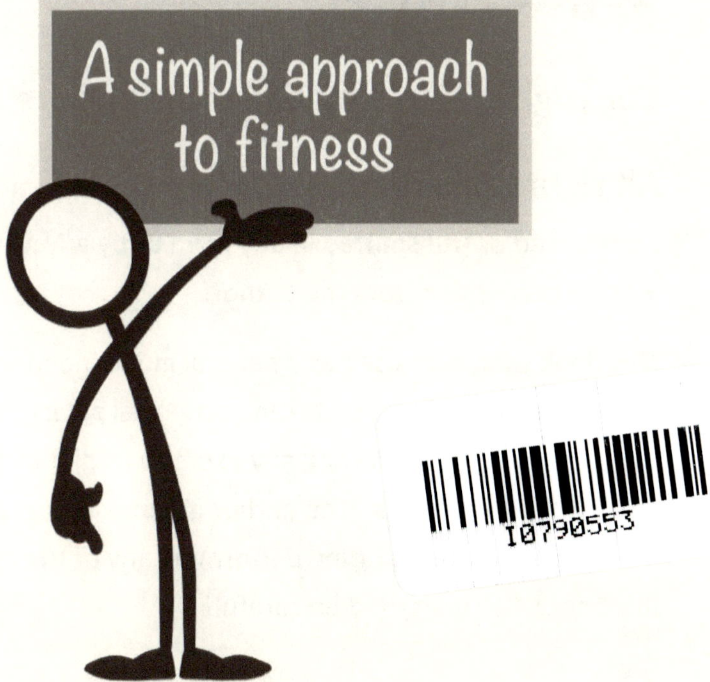

A diet and exercise philosophy for regular people

James Shropshire

Legal stuff:

Copyright ©2019 by James Shropshire

Cover design, interior layout, and illustrations by Gil Chavez

To contact Gil: GilbertoChavez.com and gil@gchavezgroup.com

ISBN: 9781794603844

LCCN: 2019901349

Follow me or contact me on Facebook @ James Shropshire

This book is dedicated to my wife and daughters.
Thanks for putting up with all of
my weirdness! I love you all!

Thanks to Rocky May for proofreading my book and
helping me to appear literate. Any mistakes were
made after he proofread it.

Thanks to Gil Chavez for the artwork and design ideas.
This book would not look anywhere near as cool
without all of your
hard work and creativity.

DISCLAIMER!!!!

Please don't sue me!!!

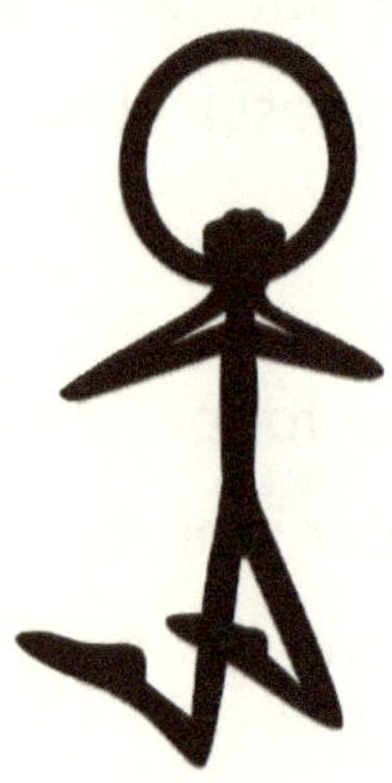

Please take this into consideration before implementing anything you read in this book into your daily routine...

I AM NOT A DOCTOR!

I AM NOT A SCIENTIST!

I DO NOT HAVE A DEGREE IN NUTRITION!

There! Now I feel much better. This book is a basic, common sense approach to getting in better shape. It is not a scientific study based on thousands of hours of research. There will not be any specific studies cited to prove any of these theories. None of these theories were originated by me. This book is about many concepts that I have tried and had success with. You may not see the same results. Everyone is different and will have a different experience. Please go and see your doctor to make sure you are healthy enough to start an exercise program. I will do my best to give credit where credit is due. I have listened to hundreds of podcasts and read numerous books on health, exercise, and nutrition. I will list the most beneficial books and podcasts in the last section if you want a more detailed and scientific outlook. Please enjoy this book as if you and I were having a conversation about health, not a specific plan that you must follow to see results.

TABLE OF CONTENTS

INTRODUCTION

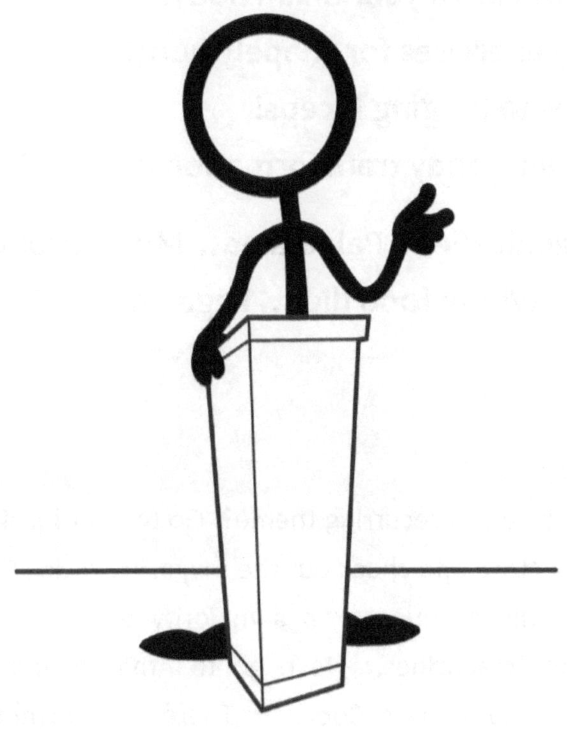

(or what will this book do for me?)

INTRODUCTION

6 pack abs! 30 days to a new you!

Two weeks to your bikini body!

3 easy exercises for shapely buns!

5 steps to bulging biceps!

Complete body transformations!

Ketogenic diet… Paleo diet… Mediterranean diet… Whole food diet… Vegan diet… Carnivore diet…

Notice a recurring theme? Go to your local grocery or book store and check out the magazine rack. These are the headlines you see on a majority of the men's and women's magazines. Next, go to Amazon and type in "Health and Fitness Books." There are currently over 60,000 titles in that category!

With that amount of information and obvious interest in the subject, you would think that we would be living in a utopian world where everyone was a supermodel or an Adonis. However, that has not been my experience. Walk around your local mall or any random outdoor festival. You will probably see a lot more people who look out of shape than people who look fit. We are getting way fatter as a nation. Heart attacks, cancer, diabetes, and many other related diseases are rising rapidly. Many doctors and experts believe this trend will continue in the future. One of the very best things you can do to improve your health is to maintain a healthy weight and exercise on a regular basis.

The reason most people don't do these things is not due to a lack of information, but an overwhelming amount of conflicting information. Every other day there is a new article that might be a direct contradiction to what you read the week before. One article says to eat lots of healthy grains. The next article says that carbs will kill you! There are studies that show that eating red meat will either give you cancer or a heart attack. However, there's another group of people that survive strictly on a meat-only diet. Supplement companies will advertise in magazines that write articles that will preach the benefits of those exact supplements (Can you say "conflict of interest"?) while trying to convince you to buy their pills or powders by showing before and after photos of amazing transformations that make you want to grab your phone and order a bottle. Unless you have a degree in nutrition, it can be difficult to decide which program to follow.

Everybody's different. There's no one diet that works for everyone.

That being said, you may be wondering why you should read yet another book about diet and exercise written by an author who doesn't even have a Ph.D. after his name. Even though I don't have any degrees, I have been studying fitness and health for a long time. Everything you read in this book is the accumulation of over 30 years of seeing what works and also what doesn't. I practice what I preach daily. Hopefully this will help to give me a little credibility. I recently had a body composition test done before taking part in a 6 week physique challenge with some friends. There were 2 main numbers that the analysis came back with that are important: 12.2 body fat percentage and 0.0 lbs. body fat mass and lean body mass.   This test was taken on a Friday after a week of clean eating to make up for my annual Labor Day weekend binge of cooking out and drinking. Having a body fat percentage of 12.2% is not too shabby for a 48 year old! The next part is the more important part. Notice how both numbers are 0.0 lbs.? That means that based on their analysis, I don't need to lose any fat or gain any muscle. Now I'm not saying that I have a perfect physique (Even though that's what the analysis said!), but it shows that what I'm doing does work. Hopefully you will apply some of things you will learn in this book and over time, achieve similar results.

I wanted to write an easy to read book with a different perspective than you see from most fitness books. This book is about adopting a new philosophy about health. You're not going to find a detailed nutrition or exercise program in this book. After 30 days of reading this book you probably won't have a six pack. If you have existing medical issues this might not cure them. I can't stress this enough: **I am not a doctor!** If I was trying to sell you a meal plan or stack of DVDs or supplements, you would be wise to ignore me. I'm just a normal guy who has struggled with body issues for my entire life and has constantly been looking for that one "miracle" diet or fitness plan or supplement that would give me those after photos I've been hoping for. I've been reading articles online and in magazines, books on nutrition, and listening to health and fitness podcasts for over 30 years. I've tried most of the diets that are listed at one time or another. I've done pretty much every kind of workout program available. There's one thing that I have noticed about almost all of the options to get in shape that are out there.

They all work! If you are consuming a standard American diet of fast food, sweets, chips, and soft drinks combined with little to no exercise, then starting any one of these programs you will begin to see results. It's almost impossible not to. Losing 5-8 pounds in your first week is very achievable. If you are able to finish the 30-day program, you could have some incredible results. You may even have that nice set of before and after photos you can post on Instagram.

Here's the problem with this whole scenario. After the 30 days are done, what next? Most of these types of programs are not sustainable. You simply can't eat and exercise like that for more than 30 days without falling off the wagon. Parties, wedding receptions, vacation, or that wine tasting you got invited to can all derail even the best of intentions. It's much more likely that you don't finish the program, which is way more common and also more likely to hurt you psychologically. Most people can tough it out the first week. You might weigh yourself and find out you lost 2-5 pounds that week. What happens the first time that you're hit with a real temptation though? Maybe it's your co-workers birthday and someone brought in a cake. Or maybe a bunch of the parents are going out for pizza and beer after the kids' soccer game. If your only motivation is looking good naked, it's going to be hard to resist. Then you wake up feeling bloated (or hungover) and then you decide to skip your morning workout. By the evening, you might be feeling a little down on yourself and have a little ice cream after dinner to help make you feel better. By the beginning of the next week, you weigh yourself again and find out you gained two pounds. A lot of people will quit after this point.

This is why I hope this book is different. I didn't get in the kind of shape I'm in by following a 30-day plan. What I did is change my philosophy about what I was trying to achieve. I changed the way that I think about eating and exercise. I stopped trying to make my appearance my primary concern, and really started focusing on my overall health. What's funny is as I focused less on trying to get abs and began focusing more on my health, I actually started to get in better shape! I'm in better shape at 48 than I was at 38. I don't beat myself up anymore if I go out for pizza and beer on a Friday night and gain 3 lbs. because I know it will be gone by Tuesday. I used to weigh myself every day and fret about any upward change in my weight or body fat percentage. Now I can use the scale to tell me how much fun I had over the weekend based on how much weight I put on. Pizza, wings, and beer taste awesome! So does a chocolate milkshake! I know if I'm forced to choose between having an underwear model physique and being able to eat my favorite foods on occasion without guilt there is no contest. (Trust me. I know from previous experience which direction I will go in!) Life is too short to deny yourself of these simple pleasures.

The reason I decided to write this book is that this is something I am very passionate about. I have seen too many people who have fallen into the trap of believing that they can't get back into shape. Too many times they have failed at programs and it's ruined their motivation to try. One of my all-time biggest mistakes I have made in my life was buying a fitness book for women for my daughter. She asked me to buy her a book to get in shape and since I'm not a woman, I went online to find something that would be right for her. Unfortunately, the book I chose had a picture of a super-ripped woman on the cover. Looking back on that decision, I feel like I did her a major disservice by picking a book that basically promoted an unachievable physique for most women as the primary goal to that book. Talk about demotivating! Most people will never get close to that kind of shape. Even the woman on the cover probably looks like that for only 5-10 days a year when she's doing a cover shoot. Most people have no desire to push themselves to that extreme. I know because I've tried. I'm known as kind of a fitness nut amongst my friends and co-workers, and have had enough people ask me for advice to realize that there needs to be a new approach to health and fitness programs.

So here is the point to this book. This is going to be a short book in comparison to a lot of health and fitness books. I'm not going to be citing a lot of scientific studies or putting a lot of footnotes to research. If you are interested in the science or more details, I will list some of the books and podcasts I got the information from. There also won't be a definitive goal or time frame you are limited to. You and I are going to focus on health, not aesthetics. I'm not trying to sell you anything. There aren't any detailed diet plans or extreme exercise programs. You're not going to be counting calories. You won't need a CrossFit membership. My goal with this book is help you to start to change your own personal philosophy. Changing the way you think about your health and what you've believed to be true for many years about diet and exercise is the first big step. This won't be a quick fix. Life is a marathon, not a sprint. You will fail at some point. Depending on where you are it might take a year or two to get to your healthy weight. Don't rush. You are going to be changing habits that might have been a lifetime in the making, and that is something that won't happen overnight. What worked for me may not work as well for you. You will have to take what you learn in this book and make it personal.

I wrote this book in 5 sections. The first section will be about my journey to come to this philosophy (I will try to keep it brief!). The point of this is to show how I've struggled and how I overcame it. The second section is all about you. Where are you at currently on this journey? What is your own definition of being in shape? What is your motivation to get healthy? This is a **HUGE** step in getting started. Knowing why you are doing this will help you at that next meeting when your boss brings in a box of donuts! There are too many benefits to being in shape to not try to get there. The next two sections will be about diet and exercise. I will explain some common misconceptions that might explain why you've had problems in the past. I will give you some basic ideas of what to eat and what to avoid. I'll also give you some exercises to help you increase your strength and flexibility. The last section will be on how to implement these ideas into your own personal philosophy that you can live with for the rest of your life. It will also include some tips on taking it to the next level. You may have a time in your life where you want to go to an extreme (beach vacation, high school reunion). You can also use this section to help jumpstart your progress. Some people are impatient and need to see immediate results to stay motivated. I use a lot of these tips to start off the New Year. A month of holiday drinks and cookies combined with a relaxed attitude towards your workouts can pack on a lot pounds quickly, especially as you get older.

My advice will be to read the first two sections, then make your list about why you want to do this in the first place. As you're reading the next three sections, take notes, start making some of the changes, and start enjoying your new healthy body. You only get one chance at this life and your health is a big factor on how that goes. You can have all of the money and possessions you could hope for, but a heart attack or cancer will take it all away. I'm not trying to live forever, but I do want to be as active as I can be for as long as I can. Being able to play with my grandkids and being healthy enough to travel in my retirement years is way more important to me now than worrying about what I might look like with my shirt off! Protect your health and you will give yourself the best chance you can to enjoy your life! Happy reading!

SECTION 1

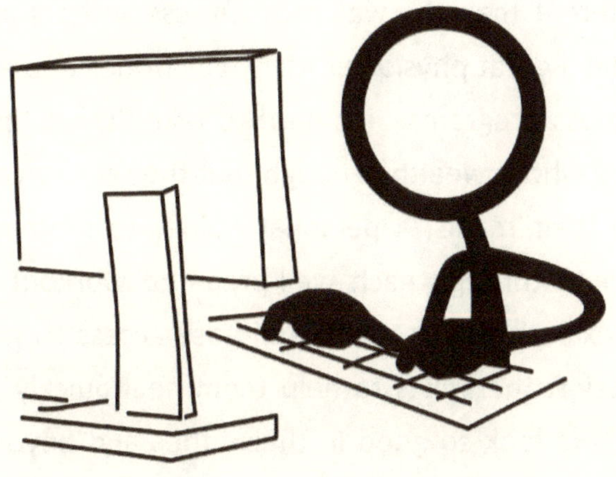

About me (or why should I listen to this guy?)

Why Should You Listen to Me?

I decided to start this book by briefly describing my journey. The average person's way of getting in shape is way different than the way most fitness authors are able to sustain a great physique. Many celebrities and athletes have fitness programs. It's hard to take fitness tips from someone who is wealthy enough that they can have a chef prepare their meals, a personal trainer to motivate and guide them through each well-prepared workout that is geared exclusively for them, and easy access to massage and physical therapists to help them heal quickly. Many male actors look so good in their fifties and beyond, not just because of good genes, but also with a little extra help from growth hormone and testosterone injections or pills. Unfortunately, I haven't reached that level of wealth yet (Come on book sales!). Here is a summary of my journey...

I was a heavy kid. It was partly due to growing up down south where most foods are breaded and fried, and partly due to my genes. My dad was a big guy, and struggled with his weight his whole life. It wasn't until sophomore year that I entered any kind of structured program. I started wrestling. This decision was both the best and worst thing I could have done. Go ask anyone who has wrestled and played any other sports and they will tell you wrestling practice is the hardest thing they've ever experienced. It gives you a great work ethic and ability to push through pain to achieve a goal. You also learn the absolute worst way to lose weight! Starvation and dehydration is how you make weight. It's also one of the worst things you can do to your metabolism. I'm fairly sure it's one of the reasons I can gain 5-7 lbs. over a single weekend of drinking and bad eating choices. After my senior year, I swore I would never diet again.

My next phase was weight lifting. Any male who grew up in the eighties looked up to Arnold Schwarzenegger and Sylvester Stallone as the ideal male physiques. I was naïve enough that I thought they actually did that through heavy lifting and supplements. I didn't realize until I was in my twenties that steroids were also used to help create those physiques. I then started working in the construction field. The problem is when you are in the prime of your life and you are burning 4000-5000 calories a day, you can pretty much eat whatever you want and still be in great shape. I would work a 10 hour day building houses, go to the YMCA gym for an hour, and then go for my favorite post-workout meal of Captain Morgan and Coke and popcorn at our favorite bar. I was built like a truck in those days.

Here's where that started to change. I got married, bought a house, and had a child. Between no longer having the time to go to the gym every day and my joints starting to hurt from all of the years of abuse in the gym and on the jobsite, my physique began to change. Eventually I had to stop lifting heavy weights, because I would be sore for 3 days after every single day of lifting. I also had multiple surgeries including a total knee replacement and partial wrist fusion to fix injuries that occurred when I was working construction.

This life experience is why I now know that you must work out **and** eat well to be in healthy shape. When I stopped lifting, I went into a depression. When your main identity is wrapped up in being the biggest guy at the party and all of a sudden you lose that, it's hard to stay motivated. You feel that if you can't work out, why bother eating healthy? I eventually got a sales job. Now I was not only not working out or eating healthy, I was also not burning the calories I was used to. I started to get softer and rounder. It took me seeing a photo of myself with slumped shoulders and a belly to shock me out of my depression.

I then began exercising again, only with much lower intensity. I also started to eat 5-6 small meals a day, which at the time was the conventional wisdom. I used a calorie tracker to monitor my daily intake and also started doing a lot more cardio. I saw almost immediate results. I dropped over 25 lbs. in about 6 months. The problem was it was a pain in the ass! Let me give you an example. My calorie counter said I needed to eat 1800 calories a day to lose a pound a week. I would have to track every meal and obsess about exact amounts to make sure I was coming in at the right amount every day. Counting every calorie you eat and having to work out every day started to take its toll. Here is where the cycle I talked about earlier started happening. I would do really well for a 2-3 week time frame, then life would happen. I'd not pack a meal, then have to stop for fast food because I was starving. I'd go to a party and drink too many beers and be hungover the next day. Now it would be time for some greasy hangover food! Skip a few workouts and eat like crap for a couple days in a row after you've turned 30 and it's amazing how far backwards you could go. I'd get discouraged and let a week go before I started back up again. I was the epitome of the yo-yo dieter.

That all changed when my brother-in-law David got a cancer diagnosis. Watching someone you've respected as a hard working self-sufficient person wither away and die from cancer after a three year battle is a real life changer. I was 39 years old when he passed away. Approaching your 40th birthday can usually be a time when you start to reflect on your own mortality anyways, but then factor in seeing someone you know die way too young will change your whole perspective on life. This was the moment when I started to develop the philosophy I now have about my body and health. I decided to stop concentrating on looking good and started to put a lot more emphasis on feeling good. If you're looking for some inspiration for being in shape as you get older, Google the Don Wildman Esquire article. This man is a real positive reinforcement for getting into and staying in good shape into your later years. He was 75 at the time of the article and could keep up with men half his age.

I started the shift from reading articles about how to get bigger muscles and six pack abs to learning more about health. I read numerous articles about how many experts believe many cancers can be traced back to the kinds of foods you eat. There is a lot of evidence that eating sugars and refined carbohydrates can increase your odds of getting certain cancers, heart attacks, and diabetes. There are also studies that show how many fruits and vegetables have anti-cancer properties. My biggest paradigm shift came from a book called "**Body for Life" by Bill Phillips**. He has a line in the book that says you need to look at food as fuel. Instead of eating for taste, I started choosing what to eat based on that food's nutritional value. Instead of doing crunches to have defined abs, I started doing planks to give my core stability and improve my posture. Instead of long cardio sessions to burn fat, I now use my elliptical machine to warm up my muscles and get my blood pumping before I start a yoga video.

Here's the main point to this story. When I was only focused strictly on my appearance, I didn't hit the goals I wanted because I didn't really want it enough. When I made the choice (and it all boils down to making that choice) to try to be as healthy as possible, a funny thing happened. I started to lose fat. Even though my muscles weren't getting noticeably bigger, by losing fat they started to be more defined. By cutting the garbage out of my diet during the week, I found it easier to bounce back from a bad weekend. My reasons for exercising went from wanting to be ripped to wanting to be like my brother-in-law's father-in-law. The guy is in his seventies and he goes for 70 mile bike rides. He actually broke his collarbone sliding headfirst into second base in his softball league! I want to be like that guy (minus the broken collarbone). In the nutrition and exercise sections, I will show you some of the things I've learned and hopefully you will be able to implement them into your own life. There is one thing you need to do before you start this journey of your own. You need to change your own philosophy. I spent hours listening to self-improvement CDs in my car by a brilliant man named Jim Rohn. The biggest takeaway I got from him was the concept of having a philosophy for every area of your life. Sticking to a strict plan or program can be almost impossible for you to maintain. Having a philosophy about eating and exercising for your long-term health will make it easier to do the right thing when your willpower may be lacking due to being tired, being under a lot of stress, or having temptation in the form of junk food.

The next section is about you. You need to take an honest look at yourself and ask yourself some hard questions. Having a "why" to being in shape is more important than learning "how" to get into shape. Once you have the reasons to get into shape, the how becomes way easier. Let's look at some possible reasons to get you started.

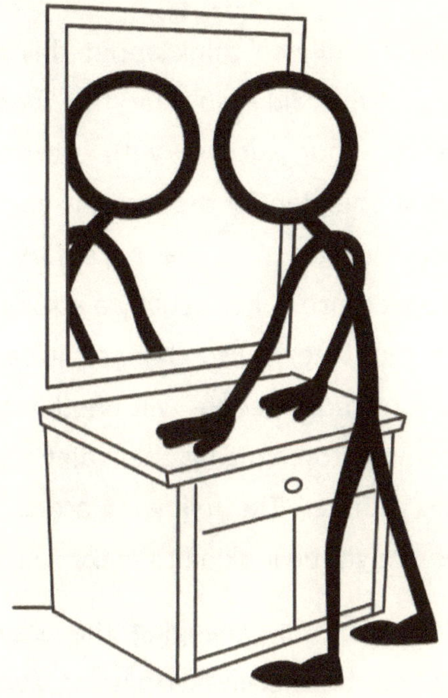

About you (or why should I listen to this guy?)

Why Are You Reading This Book?

Take a while to think about this question before answering. Why did you buy this book? It is very important for your success with starting any type of program that you identify the reasons you would consider making the changes that are necessary. As I learned, physical appearance is not usually a strong enough reason by itself to motivate you to change. It can be a powerful motivator, but most people will need more than that to actually commit to changing their diet and incorporating an exercise routine. The following are some more of the reasons you might be looking to make a change.

My reason for changing the way I think about fitness was my brother-in-law passing away from cancer. Maybe you have had a similar experience with a friend or family member. Once you get into your forties you start knowing or hearing a lot more about people getting cancer, having a heart scare, or getting a variety of health diagnosis that you didn't think about in your thirties. Take some time and Google obesity and cancer, obesity and diabetes, and the like. What you will find will be mind-blowing. I was going to write an entire paragraph on all of the percentages of how being obese can lead to various diseases, but then I realized I would have to put footnotes to back all of those claims. I'm way too lazy to do that! Go do your own research. It will be more impactful for you to take the time to do it yourself. Just the risk of disease alone should be enough to make some changes.

You might have just had a major life change. Getting divorced is probably one of the biggest reasons people might start going to the gym. Whether it's trying to get back in shape as you begin to enter the dating pool for the first time in years, looking for a way to meet new people, or just trying something new, going to the gym is many peoples' way of coping. Maybe it's an injury that put you on the shelf for way longer than you had anticipated. There are many valid reasons to start trying to improve your health.

I believe the most powerful motivator is how your health relates to how good your life is. The older I get, the more the thought of being old terrifies me! Now I'm not talking about being afraid of dying or wanting to live forever. I am afraid of becoming fragile and unable to take care of myself. I don't want to become the feeble old man who can't cut his own grass, open a jar, or to run around chasing his grandkids through the sprinkler. Most people know about someone's parent who fell and broke their hip in their seventies who never left the hospital because they wound up dying from complications of the surgery. You probably have no problem thinking up an image of an old person hunched over a walker struggling to walk up a hill. That's scary. Having someone go through the long and painful process of dying of cancer, stroke, or heart disease can be a huge wake-up call to start changing your own lifestyle. Everything is cumulative. You don't have a heart attack after you have eaten that first cheeseburger. Most heart attacks can be traced back to years of neglecting to exercise and not eating healthy. Ever hear the expression "Use it or lose it"? If you don't exercise, your body will start to atrophy. Your muscles start to shrink, your sense of balance will start to go away, and you will start to get aches and pains even if you've never had any actual physical trauma. Years of poor nutrition causes obesity which will lead to many other health-related issues. Arteries don't get clogged overnight! You should be selfish. Use your own interests as a reason for change.

The next reason could be how your health relates to your loved ones. I want to be here for my family. I want to be able to travel with my wife after my kids have moved out and started their own families. I want to help my daughters when they move furniture into their first home. I want to be able to hold my grandkids and run around with them. I don't ever want to have to plan a family vacation around my own limitations. I truly believe you owe it to your spouse to try to be as healthy as possible. If you are committing to someone to spend the rest of your life with them, you should do your best to make that as easy on them as possible. Being in shape will also improve your sex life. For men, being in shape makes for better blood flow, which helps make for better erections. I don't want to ever have to take Viagra unless it's just to try to make sex better, not because I can't perform. Being confident in your body will also make you more comfortable in the bedroom. The better that your sex life is, the better your relationship will be. Sex is the most fun thing you can do for free, so you might as well do it for as long as possible! Exercise is also proven to release the endorphins that help improve your mood and your sleep. Sounds like a good reason to me to exercise!

You also owe it to your children as well. Both of my wife's parents died young. She was only 22 when her mom passed away. Her main complications came from years of smoking. I know that my wife would have benefitted from having her mom there to help her plan our wedding. Raising children would have also been a little easier with a little motherly advice. My daughters will have a much better life if my wife is there to guide them through their young adult life. I'd like to stick around as well. Helping them to pick out their first house, make career decisions, or fix a leaky sink feels like a good way to contribute to them having the best life possible.

That's a powerful reason to try to stick around. Maybe her mom would have passed away before her time without the smoking addiction, but it definitely didn't help. Hopefully you never picked up this nasty habit, but if so you need to quit NOW! Smoking and excessive sugar consumption are two of the worst things you can do to your body. You should be smarter than that.

Another strong motivator may having nothing to do with health. Maybe you have a bucket list that includes running a marathon, climbing Mt. Everest, or hiking in the Grand Canyon. When your children get older you start looking to do more things for yourself. My boss just turned 50 this year. He has a similar mindset to me and also has a very competitive side. He plays soccer with guys that are in their twenties and has been competing in Spartan races for the last couple of years. This gives him a reason to train that is not related to his appearance or longevity. He simply wants to compete! He also doesn't want to embarrass himself against the young guys. That's all the more reason to not eat that donut and have a handful of almonds instead.

Last, but not least, is your physical appearance. There is nothing wrong with being proud about the type of body you have, as long as you're not obnoxious about it. People consider vanity to be a selfish trait, but I don't think it is in most cases. If you are comparing yourself to other people to put them down then that would be a different story. People should be proud of their achievements. I'm 48. It's a lot harder to be in shape at 48 than it was at 28. When someone guesses my age as 40, it makes me feel good. Eating healthy and exercising will also make your skin look more youthful. Various people over the years have asked me for help on getting in shape or nutrition advice which is why I decided to write this book in the first place. Now, I'm not "ripped" or "shredded" or have huge muscles, but I still wear the same size jeans I wore in high school. I'm pretty lean and have big enough muscles that I still look like I could take care of myself if necessary. There's nothing wrong with being proud of the work you did and the sacrifices you made to achieve the physique you have. Everyone is a little vain in their own way. Most women, regardless of their shape, will still put on make-up and do their hair before they go out. Most men still want to feel like they could step up in case of an emergency and be able to protect their loved ones. The flip side to appearance is that it's also the best indicator of progress. You can't really tell 100% how much more healthy you are because a lot of it is preventative medicine. You can definitely tell if your pants are getting looser or if you need to move up a belt loop. Buying new clothes that fit your new physique is a great reinforcement to continuing your health journey.

Take some time to figure out why you are doing this. Writing down the reasons on a piece of paper helps reinforce this in your own brain. You don't need to look at this list daily, but looking at it periodically will help your motivation, especially if you've slipped up (which will happen). After you figure out the why, then it becomes about figuring out the how. The next three sections will help you to make a new plan for improvement. I believe that diet is way more important than exercise, but they both will feed off of each other. If you had a really good workout in the morning, you're much more likely to skip the junk food and eat something healthy. If you have a healthy dinner and a good night's sleep you will be much more likely to have a good workout the next day. The more you continue this cycle, the better you will look and feel, which will make it easier to stick with it. It's all about momentum. Let's get started with learning the basic concepts about nutrition in the next section.

SECTION 3

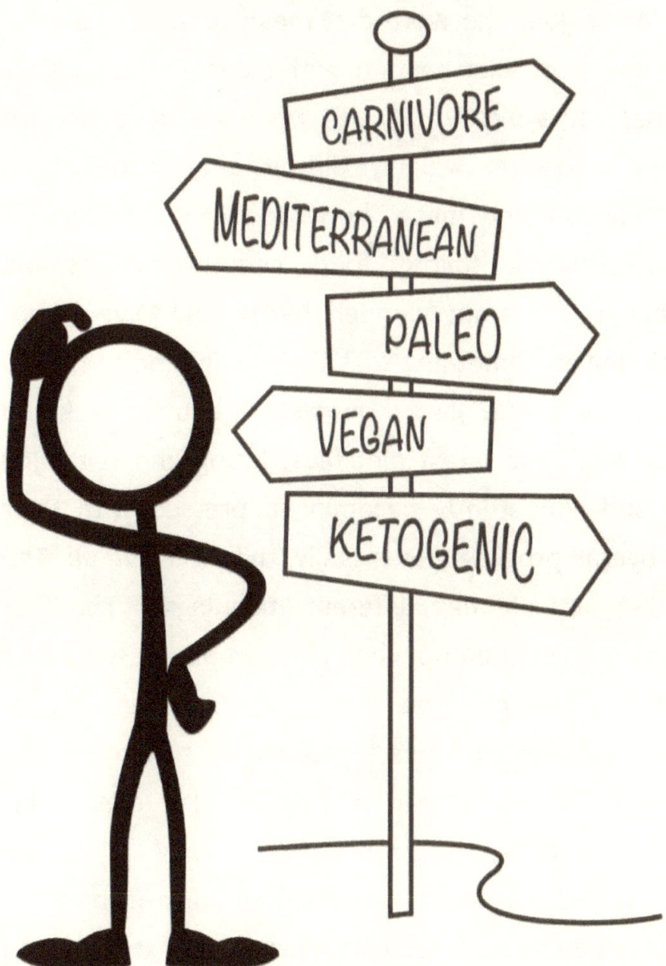

About diet (80% focus)

About Diet

What does the word diet mean to you? To most people, the word diet has a negative connotation. It's a word that you typically only use when you've gotten fat and need to lose the weight. Nobody gets excited about committing to a new diet. The word diet is synonymous with restricting your favorite foods, counting calories, and being hungry. Is it any wonder that people have a hard time sticking to something that they really don't want to do in the first place? Many people will bounce back and forth between the latest diet fads, losing and regaining weight and consistently becoming depressed with their lack of overall progress. Eventually, they will give up. The word diet actually has different meanings. The first definition that popped up when I looked up the word diet was "the kinds of food that a person, animal, or community habitually eats." Examples would be the Vegan diet, Mediterranean diet, and Paleo diet. This definition would be the proper way to think about the word diet. The way most people would think of the word diet would be the next two examples. The next definition was "a special course of food to which one restricts oneself, either for losing weight or for medical reasons." The example given was "I'm going on a diet". Not exactly as exciting as saying you're going on a vacation! As a verb, the definition came up as "restrict oneself to small amounts or special kinds of food in order to lose weight." The example given for that was "It's difficult to diet". That seems to be what a majority of peoples' perception of dieting is. That's why I think that changing your philosophy about how you eat will help more than trying to stick to a "diet." My personal philosophy about how I eat is much simpler than the average diet. I eat as healthy as I can for as many meals as I can so that when I go off of the rails, I don't feel guilty. Let's say you eat 3 meals a day for a week. That's 21 meals. If you eat 3 cheat meals a week, you are eating healthy meals 85% of the time. That's good enough to help keep you in good shape for the rest of your life. I also try to eat as many foods that have as few of ingredients as possible. I try to get a variety of healthy fats, protein, and fiber in every regular meal. I avoid eating processed foods that have ingredients that I don't know or can't pronounce. I avoid sugar and other refined carbs that will spike my insulin levels and make me hungry again a few hours later. I have brainwashed myself into looking at sugar as poison. I don't worry about counting calories because if I'm getting fat, protein, and fiber in my meal, I will get full without overeating. Try this experiment. Go all day without eating until dinner. You should be pretty hungry at this point. Now try eating an apple. That first apple will be delicious, especially if you've kicked your sugar addiction. (More on kicking your sugar addiction later.) Now eat another apple. It will still taste good, but not as good as the first. By the time you finish the third apple, you will be full and you won't have the urge to continue eating apples. Now try the same experiment on the next day, only do it with pizza. You will find it that it's much easier to continue eating junk food long after your calorie requirements have been met. I can't tell you how many times I've been stuffed on pizza, only to reach for "one" more piece! Sometimes that one extra piece turns into two or three extra pieces until I've become uncomfortably full. The point to this is that it is virtually impossible for you to overeat with healthy foods. It's extremely easy for you to overindulge in your favorite foods. I have three different types of eating days. The first day would be a perfect day. I would have eaten nothing but a good combination of fruits and vegetables for nutrients and fiber, healthy fats and oils, and some form of meat or organic plant based protein powder for my protein needs. That happens 3-4 days a week. The second day would be 1-2 days a week and would involve eating 1-2 perfect meals, but sometimes I don't have a chance to pack enough healthy food. I then might stop and grab a Muscle Milk and a bag of almonds. If I can't eat healthy, I try to go for macros and make sure that I'm getting fat, fiber and protein even if the source isn't the greatest. The third type of day would be the day that I have a cheat meal which could also be 1-2 days. On that day it's really all about keeping my calories low. Everything I will eat up until that point will include healthy protein and fiber with lower fat. 25% of the calories that you get from eating protein are burned to digest the protein. You will want lots of fiber to push everything through your system quicker and also to make you feel full. I will typically eat a large salad within a few of hours of going out if I know I'm going to be eating heavy foods with dessert and drinking alcohol. If you can follow this type of eating pattern, you will start to see results almost immediately.

The reason many people have trouble getting in the kind of shape they want to be in is due to a lot of misinformation about food and how your body metabolizes what you eat. We've been told for years that calorie restriction is the way to lose weight. Eat less, exercise more. Create a calorie deficit and the weight has to come off, right? First of all, all calories are not equal. A 100- calorie pack of almonds will do different things to your body than a 100-calorie pack of cookies. The almonds have healthy fat, protein, and fiber to give you energy and help to keep you full until your next meal. The cookies are full of refined carbohydrates and sugar that won't fill you up and will actually cause you to either eat another pack, or spike your insulin levels so that you are hungry an hour later. There is a whole science that is devoted to making foods with the perfect blend of unhealthy fats (vegetable and soybean oils), sugar, artificial colors and flavors, and other chemicals to make their "foods" addicting. Look on the nutrition facts label of most 100-calorie packs of cookies and other treats. Most of them will have a least 2-3 different versions of sweeteners. Second, how do you know how many calories you will need each day? Every day is different.

Let me give you two examples from my own life. I work in sales. Every other Friday I have the day off (I work every Saturday). If its summer, I'll usually get up and have a cup of coffee with a splash of heavy cream while my dogs eat. I'll then go on an hour-long walk with them to get them their daily exercise. Depending on where I'm at with my workout schedule, I may do a 30 minute strength workout. After I finish, I will go out and cut my grass and trim the bushes. If I'm lucky, I might go out for a round of golf. I'll try to take my dogs for another walk and then maybe go for a walk in the evening with my wife. Lots of movement, lots of calories burned. Now take the following Sunday. I'll usually run 2-3 appointments on Saturday which doesn't leave me much time for a workout or long walk. Then I might go out for a big dinner and drinks with my wife or go hang out with some friends for drinks. The next day I usually have a food and alcohol hangover (turning 40 really sucks for the amount of booze or heavy food you can consume and still function the next day!). Sundays usually involve less movement than Fridays.

I will also still be digesting and metabolizing all of the garbage I put into my body the day before.

The problem with most diets is they are based on you eating the same amount of calories every day based on some table that uses your age, sex, weight, and weight loss goals. Everyone burns calories different. We all know that one person (who we hate!) who can eat whatever they want and not gain a pound. When I go on our every-other year beach vacation with my wife's family, I will gain anywhere from 8-12 pounds in a week. I'm definitely not that person! Trying to figure out the exact amount of calories your body requires on a daily basis is pretty much impossible. The other problem is most people don't truly know what is healthy and what isn't. Let's take a look at a normal day in the average adult's diet.

Many people start with a cup or two of coffee. They either put milk and sugar or some type of flavored creamer to sweeten their coffee. A "healthy" breakfast of orange juice, a packet of instant oatmeal or cereal and they are off to work. Because of all of the sugar they get from the creamer, juice, and breakfast they are feeling a burst of energy to get their day started. However, it is usually short- lived. Because they didn't get any healthy fat and protein, their energy is soon gone. Their insulin levels have spiked to help metabolize the sugar. Their body is not fat adapted, so when the sugar is burned up their body doesn't know how to burn their own fat for energy so they start getting hungry again. Using sugar and carbs for energy is like having a bonfire with small sticks and gasoline. To keep the fire burning, you constantly have to keep adding sticks and gas to restart it. Becoming fat adapted is like using charcoal and big logs. Once it's started, it will burn for a long time without needing additional fuel. Now you're getting hungry again and lunch is hours away. They will have a "healthy" granola bar (sugar and refined carbs) and then start the cycle all over again or they suffer until lunch. Lunch may be a sandwich and chips or leftovers from the night before washed down with a soda. After a couple of cycles of highs and lows, they start getting the afternoon crash. Here comes the coffee or an energy drink to save the day! By the time they get home, they're too tired to get in a workout and will settle for whatever takeout they decided to pick up for dinner with a beer or a glass of wine to drink. For dessert they decide to have a low-fat 100 calorie ice cream sandwich. After 10 years of this type of lifestyle, you can easily put on 10- 30 pounds of pure fat, not to mention the 5-10 pounds of muscle you may have lost. To add insult to injury, the fatter you get, the easier it is to keep putting on the pounds. The heavier you get, the harder it is to get motivated to exercise. Living this type of lifestyle will increase your odds of getting cancer, diabetes, having a major heart attack or stroke, or shortening your overall amount of quality years before you get too old to do anything. That's not the place you want to be at, looking back on what might have been.

Let's take a look at why this type of day is so bad for you. You are waking up with an empty stomach and you're also dehydrated. Over the course of the night you have digested all of the food that you consumed the day before. Your body has been in healing mode as you've slept. When you put sugar and milk or creamer in your body as its first form of calories, you are literally telling your body not to burn your own fat for energy. Your body will always find the easiest way to do things. It's a lot easier for your body to access the immediate dose of sugar and turn off any potential for fat burning. Many people are looking for the quick fix when it comes to losing weight. They think making a major change will help them, but it is the little things that count. Take your favorite coffee creamer. Most flavored creamer has at least 5 grams of sugar per tablespoon. Next time you make a cup of coffee, actually measure out the creamer with a tablespoon. The first time I tried this, I realized that I was using way more than one tablespoon. Even using only one tablespoon as an example, if you only have one cup of coffee a day for 365 days, that's **1825** grams of sugar a year you've consumed instead of drinking your coffee black or using some heavy whipping cream in place of the creamer. That amount of sugar alone could cause you to gain 2-3 pounds of pure fat in one year. Now let's look at that glass of orange juice. Seems healthy, right? Look at the label on your orange or apple juice. There is almost as much sugar in 12 ounces of juice as there is in the same 12 ounces of Coke. Now there is also a decent amount of sugar in an orange or apple. The difference is you will get some fiber from eating the fruit which helps to lower the insulin spike that you receive from the sugar. Then if you add in instant oatmeal or some cereal with milk, you have turned your body into a sugar burning machine. The problem with most "healthy" cereal is that even though it's fortified with vitamins, your body just isn't going to absorb most of those vitamins because they aren't in a natural form. I know I said there would be no calorie counting in the introduction, but a helpful tool for beginners would be to use a calorie tracker for a couple of days. Most calorie trackers will give you a detailed breakdown of the fat, carbs, protein, fiber and sugar. I personally have used the Livestrong tracker. It was extremely helpful in letting me know how unhealthy some of the foods I was eating really were. You might be surprised at how many grams of sugar that you consume in one day. Now let's examine the unnecessary midmorning snack. One of my favorite books that I strongly recommend reading is **"The Primal Blueprint" by Mark Sisson.** His book will take you through the typical day of how our ancestors ate and exercised. Our bodies have not evolved to be constantly eating meals. When you eat three full meals and a couple of snacks a day, your body spends all day long digesting food. It takes a lot of energy to digest food. Think of all the additional energy you would have if you weren't going through that process all day long! Many times when people need a snack, it's because they are either feeling bored or they are dehydrated. The next time you feel like a snack, get up and walk to the water cooler and drink a full glass of water. By the time you get back to your desk, you probably won't be hungry anymore. I hope you are starting to get the picture. A whole wheat bread with processed lunch meat sandwich with chips and a Coke aren't going to supply you with any long term energy either. It's time to change the way you think about food and also the way you think about how often you need to eat.

One of the biggest problems is most people think you need carbs for energy and that fat is the enemy. If you grew up in the eighties, you were brainwashed into believing that fat was bad for you, especially saturated fats. Everything that you saw was labeled fat-free. You were told you should drink skim milk. Instead of having a nutritious breakfast of scrambled eggs, you would have a bowl of Wheaties. People starting getting busier, so instead of meat and vegetables for dinner, we started eating Hamburger Helper. Weight Watchers and Nutrisystem became the go-to for people for dieting. If you needed a snack you could grab a Slim-Fast. Here's what happened. People stayed fat! You replaced a meal with a can of Slim-Fast, but then you were starving an hour later. Then came the big diet pill craze. Anyone remember the prescription drug Phen-fen? That worked really well for fat loss. It also had an interesting array of unwanted side effects including heart attacks, stroke, and birth defects! The problem was that you were attacking the symptom, not the cause of the weight gain in the first place. If you don't know what to eat and why, what do you do when you're done with the meal plan?

Here's a realistic way you can eat for health and long term fitness. You should incorporate as many one-ingredient foods as possible. It's important to eat healthy fats with every meal. Fat will make you fuller for longer which will result in eating less over all. Even saturated fat has multiple benefits, especially for men. It is a key component in hormone regulation. Many people worry about eating eggs for the saturated fat and cholesterol content. There are many studies that show that eating cholesterol doesn't directly affect your cholesterol levels. Eating saturated fat is bad for you only if you're eating it with high amounts of sugar and refined carbs. You shouldn't be eating those anyways! The following is a list of healthy fats that you should be eating: eggs, fatty cuts of grass fed beef- 85/15 ground beef, ribeye etc., nuts and seeds (raw if possible, dry roasted if not), olive, coconut, avocado, and macadamia oils, avocados, nut butters (only ingredients should be nuts and salt), salmon, tins of sardines or mackerel, grass-fed butter, and hard cheeses (no processed cheese foods!) Just remember that fat has more calories per gram than protein or carbohydrates. Eating a handful of nuts is a good snack. Eating the entire bag may be a bit too much!

You should always try to eat a decent amount of protein and fiber as well. Protein contains amino acids which help to preserve muscle. You may not want to look like a body builder, but maintaining your muscles will help you as you age. There are multiple studies that say you should get more protein as you get older to fight the natural loss of muscle from aging. You can get plenty of fiber from eating lots of vegetables, nuts, and beans. Eating fiber can help slow down the digestive process so that you avoid spikes in insulin and to help you feel fuller for longer. Vegetables, nuts, and beans also do contain carbohydrates. I'm not against all carbs. I'm against refined carbs. Fruits are okay to have but I would limit most fruits on a regular basis. Apples and berries are fine because they will have fiber to offset the sugar, but oranges, grapes and bananas are unnecessary unless you just want one for the taste. Feel free to eat fresh fruit when it is season. There's not too many desserts that will taste as good as a fresh peach or strawberries from the local farmer's market. If you live in an area that doesn't have a lot of fresh fruit to pick from, buy organic frozen fruit. They are great for a smoothie or to add to some plain yogurt.

You may have grown up in a family where every meal had to have a side of rice, pasta, noodles, or potatoes. That's one of the first things I hear from people is that they can't give up pasta or bread. These foods really don't have that much taste. It's the combination of pasta, rice, or noodles with whatever sauce you choose to have with it that makes it taste so good. Baked potatoes are okay as long as you eat them sparingly. Try to stay away from white carbs. Those are the ones that cause the most trouble. Replace them with additional vegetables. You can get almost all of the vitamins and minerals you need from eating a wide variety of vegetables and meat. Mix it up. One meal you can have salmon, the next you can have grilled chicken. Some of your salads may have spinach, others may have romaine or kale. It's never been easier to get organic produce at a reasonable price. Most grocery stores now have big containers of spinach, spring mix, and many other organic vegetables. I'm a firm believer in trying to buy organic when it comes to produce. It's simply better for your body. I'm also a big believer in organic, free range and grass-fed meats. Those can be a lot pricier, but you can find healthy options. Grass-fed organic ground beef can be found at most grocery stores, including Target and Walmart. Organic eggs are also not that expensive. Spend the money to get healthier food if you're able to. Buy what you can afford though. If you can't afford organic meats, regular meat is still better for you in the long run than a meal of processed junk.

One of the best things you can do for your health is to break your sugar addiction. Many people tell me that no matter how hard they try they just can't quit bread or sweets. They feel like they don't have any willpower when it comes to these foods. I get it. A hamburger tastes better when you eat it on a pretzel roll than when you eat it without the bun. Part of the reason that you have this problem though has nothing to do with the taste. You are literally addicted to either the sugar that's in the product, or the sugar that it will turn into when your body digests it. What you need to do is eliminate all of the sugars and refined carbs from your diet until you break this addiction. You will need to detox from sugar! You can literally have both a physical and mental addiction to sugar. Take a minute and think about what the first major event of your life was (other than actually being born!). If you're like a lot of people, it was probably your first birthday. You were put in a chair in front of a room full of people who were singing to you. Then you had a piece of cake put in front of you and you were actually encouraged to pick up the cake with your hands and shove it in your mouth! Everyone even laughed and applauded when you got the frosting all over yourself. You just received your first lesson in gluttony! From that point on, almost every major event had some form of sugary treat. For your birthdays you had a party where you had cake and ice cream. On the first day of school you may have been taken out for a doughnut. At campfires you had s'mores. After going sledding you have a cup of hot cocoa with marshmallows. Is it any wonder then that almost all people associate sugar with pleasure? That's why it can be so hard to break this addiction. Here's how you'll realize you're addicted. Most people that try to completely detox from sugar will actually get a cold that can last anywhere from 2-3 days up to 2-3 weeks depending on how much sugar they used to eat. It's called the keto flu, which is named after the ketogenic diet. I had a kid I work with who was having a hard time losing weight even though he played soccer three times a week and also worked out at the gym. I told him to cut out all of the sugar he normally ate. He was sick for well over a week. He kept telling me he had the flu. I told him to tough it out. After he got through with his "sickness", he told me that not only did he start dropping the pounds without adding any more workouts, he also wasn't craving the bad foods he was eating before that was keeping him from being at the weight he wanted to be. I **highly** recommend that you give this a try. Commit to going at least 2-3 weeks without eating any sugar, including all fruits, breads, pasta, noodles, rice, alcohol, etc. Two weeks is not really a long time in the grand scheme of things. It will really help. If you try to lose fat and get back into shape without doing a sugar detox you are making it much harder on yourself. It's like trying to drive your car with the parking brake on. Give yourself the best chance to succeed. It will also change your taste buds. When you're not a sugar junkie, a healthy apple or a small bowl of blueberries will taste really good! I also like to take grapes or cut up watermelon and freeze them. It's a delicious and refreshing summer treat. Every once in a while, you will probably get a craving for something sweet other than fruit. Cocoa and cinnamon roasted almonds are my go-to when I need a little bit of sweet after a meal. Now I know they will have some chemicals in them that I would rather not consume, but if eaten occasionally I don't think that it's doing too much harm overall. A couple of squares of dark chocolate with almonds and sea salt is also delicious. Try to get at least 70% dark chocolate and watch the sugar. When I'm craving some ice cream, I will make a protein shake that consists of almond milk, a scoop of chocolate protein powder, a spoonful of peanut butter, and a few ice cubes blended. It's not as good as an ice cream milkshake, but it is close enough to satisfy my craving.

Are you starting to get the idea about how important your diet really is? There are a lot of options for healthy and tasty meals. You can also go online and get many recipes for home-made salad dressings, marinades, and seasonings you can make at home. My wife is a big fan of using Pinterest recipes. Last year she got on a big salad kick where they had a lot of recipes for salads that were an entire meal. They were both delicious and filling. The best part is they were also easy to make and nutritious. This year it's been single pan dinners. Meat, vegetables, potatoes, olive oil, and spices are the only ingredients. Please don't make the mistake of thinking that healthy meals have to be bland! Use your creativity (or Pinterest) to come up with some great meals for you and your family. The best part is you can control what goes into your body.

You can use the same principles when you go out to eat. Almost every decent restaurant will have a meat and vegetables offering. If not, order off the menu. Most places won't have a problem modifying the meals. We go out for lunch after our sales meetings. I usually order some combination of beef, fish, or chicken with a side or two of vegetables. If I order a steak salad, I have them make it with no dressing and ask for some olive oil and red wine vinegar. Many time my younger salesmen will order the burger and fries, then comment on how they wish they could eat as healthy as I do! It's a matter of making that your philosophy. It's easy to cheat on your diet. It's harder to go back on a commitment you made to yourself. Here's the best part though. Sometimes I will have the cheeseburger and fries! Life is way too short to not be able to sample the wings sometimes. Just be sure to not do it often. Enjoy your cheat meal. If I've eaten a large cheat meal around 2-3 in the afternoon, I usually won't eat a normal dinner then to make up for it. A handful of raw almonds and an apple with a glass of water should be enough to tide me over until the morning. I believe that cheat meals are very important to being able to stick to a healthy overall philosophy of eating. Change your thinking about cheat meals. Call them reward meals! Consider them a reward for having done a good job during the week of eating well. You will actually enjoy these foods more if you only eat them on occasion. There's something interesting about reward meals and trying to get into shape. As you start to see results, you actually start to crave reward meals less. If you've dropped 2-3 pounds from Monday morning to Friday morning, you might be less inclined to have a reward meal on Friday night! Overeating on occasion is also good for you when you've been eating healthy for a long period of time. It can help to reset your metabolism. After eating healthy for a few weeks you may start to reach a plateau. It's a two steps forward one step back approach to losing weight. It will also help reinforce good eating habits during the day when you know you will be eating poorly that evening. If I know that I will be going out for dinner and drinks then I will make sure to have a healthy day to compensate. I also use the same approach when it comes to alcohol. I believe people just get used to drinking in certain situations. You automatically order a glass of wine or beer when you go out to eat. I try to limit my drinking to the weekend. It's just another reward for a good week of eating healthy. If you are drinking on a daily basis you might want to re-think that. Alcohol is poison to your body. Why do you think you feel so bad the next day after a fun evening? Your body has to stop everything productive and focus on metabolizing the sugars from the alcohol. Your sleep will begin to suffer and you may make poor food choices the next day. Save it for once or twice a weekend. The same thing applies though to drinking as it does to reward meals on your plan. If some friends I haven't seen in a while are getting together for drinks, I won't hesitate to join them. Feel free to indulge every once in a while, just be sure to make up for it afterwards.

I also want to focus on what you drink. This is where many people are sabotaging their diet without really thinking about it. I shouldn't have to inform you about how unhealthy soft drinks are, even diet soda. It's really made up of nothing but chemicals and artificial sweeteners and colors. I listen to the Joe Rogan podcast daily and one of my favorite phrases of his has to do with how people are obsessed with "mouth pleasure". You're not 5 years old anymore! I've heard of many people who lost 10-20 pounds by simply cutting out their 2-3 a day habit of soda or sugary coffee drinks. I primarily drink water, green tea, and coffee. You can make a pitcher of water with lemon or lime slices, some cucumbers, and a few mint leaves to give it a better flavor. Experiment with different combinations. You can also drink mineral water with a splash of fresh lemon or lime juice if you're still craving some carbonation. To make my green tea taste better, I add a peppermint or cinnamon tea bag. It gives it just enough flavor. I use a splash of heavy cream and sometimes a dash of cinnamon in my coffee. Does it taste like the sugary drink you get from Starbucks? Hell no! You have to put it into perspective though. It will take you 10 minutes to drink your coffee. That 10 minutes can affect how your body is going to function for the next 2-3 hours. Make the smart choice. I do like to have my coffee with some hazelnut creamer on Sunday morning. It's my mini-cheat that I actually really look forward to. It tastes way better drinking it only one day than it would if I drank it every day. The same thing applies to soft drinks. About once or twice a month I find myself craving a fountain Diet Coke. Because I have that so rarely, I don't feel bad about indulging every once in a while. The only other thing I drink is kombucha. There is a lot of research about the many benefits of probiotics for your gut that can be found in fermented foods. Eating sauerkraut, yogurt, and kimchi and drinking kombucha and kefir are great ways to help out your gut health which can affect your overall health. Just be careful to watch the sugar content.

The last part of this section is about not eating. Many of you may have heard about intermittent fasting. This is where you eat in limited time frame. The most popular time frame is 8 hours of eating followed by 16 hours of fasting. Your body spends a lot of energy digesting food when it would be better off using that energy to repair cells. After your body has fully digested the food that you have consumed, it will start the process of healing. It's easy to look at fasting as something that might be too-next level for what you are trying to achieve. I hope you will reconsider that thought. People look at doing a one day fast as something that is extreme, but there are many people on this earth that will go a day without eating on a regular basis due to lack of food. You may have to ease slowly into fasting that long, but the benefits are well worth it. Start off with a simple 12 hour fast. Eat dinner at 7p.m. then don't eat anything until 7 a.m. The next day either eat dinner sooner or eat breakfast later by an hour. Eventually you will work your way up to 16 hours. By limiting your eating window, you may naturally eat less. The biggest benefit is that it teaches you that there isn't anything wrong with being a little hungry! If you are eating every 2-3 hours, you will start to become hungry every 2-3 hours. If you go past that window, you can start to develop that ugly "hangry" feeling. Feeling this way may cause you to make poor choices due to whatever food is near you when this happens. The more you try fasting, the easier it becomes. Fasting when you are fat adapted is way easier than if you are a sugar junkie. You'll realize that the feeling that you ascribe to being "starving" really isn't that big of a deal. Have you ever had a mild headache? It may bother you for a little bit but not enough to take anything for it. What's funny about that is if you get involved in any type of activity that you enjoy, you eventually don't think about your headache. It will be the same thing with being slightly hungry. I will try to fast every Monday. I'll eat dinner on Sunday evening, then I won't have anything to eat until dinner on Monday evening and do a full day fast. Occasionally I won't eat until breakfast on Tuesday. It all depends on how I feel. I know now what true hunger is. This helps in two ways. It lets me know if I'm truly hungry and really need food or if I'm just bored or dehydrated. It can also help to develop the mental fortitude so I won't make bad food choices when I am truly hungry or when I'm faced with a temptation. How many times have you not been hungry, but then you see a commercial for some food that made your mouth water and now you're starving? It has happened to everyone. What happens if you don't get up and grab something to eat? Usually, that hungry feeling will pass. You weren't really hungry to begin with. I do a lot of travelling for work where I may have an appointment in one city, then have to drive an hour to get to my next appointment. Sometimes the appointments can overlap if one goes longer than expected. I won't have time to stop and grab lunch. With this self-discipline gained by fasting, I can either suffice with a bag of almonds and a bottle of water from a gas station or I just don't eat. **I'm ok with being hungry!** By the time I've started my next appointment I've already forgotten about that hungry feeling. This is very liberating. It can allow me to get more done than in the past where I felt it necessary to eat every 3 hours. You can do the same thing with practice. The reason I like doing it on Monday because I usually overeat and drink alcohol at least once or twice during the weekend. This gives my body a chance to repair any damage I may have done. Make sure to have at least one really healthy meal before starting the fast. If you have a reward meal on Sunday night, hold off on fasting until Tuesday morning. I've been doing this for so long now that I'm not even hungry until at least noon on Mondays. It's like my body knows that it need a break. The best part is the longer you stick to eating healthy foods and fasting, the more your body will actually crave healthy foods. I now prefer a big bowl of greens with a cut up chicken breast, assorted vegetables, sunflower seeds, blue cheese crumbles, avocado, and a healthy salad dressing to a big helping of lasagna and garlic bread. I definitely feel better after that kind of meal as well.

Here's what you need to do. Take a good hard look at your daily eating habits. Take a week and write down everything you eat. Using a calorie counter is very helpful for this. There are many apps you can put on your phone to make this as easy as possible. You probably already know what you're doing wrong. This stuff is all common sense. As I've referenced before, you need to look at the food you put into your body as fuel. Good food will make your body run like a finely tuned machine. It is the easiest way to put the odds in your favor to avoid serious diseases, as well as turning your body into a fat burner, not a sugar burner. Eating poorly will make you sluggish, unmotivated, and old before your time. I truly believe that your nutrition is 80% of the equation to having a healthy body. It's not enough though to only eat well. You will also need to get moving! The more you combine diet and exercise the better your results. The exercise section will help to get you started in the right direction.

SECTION 4

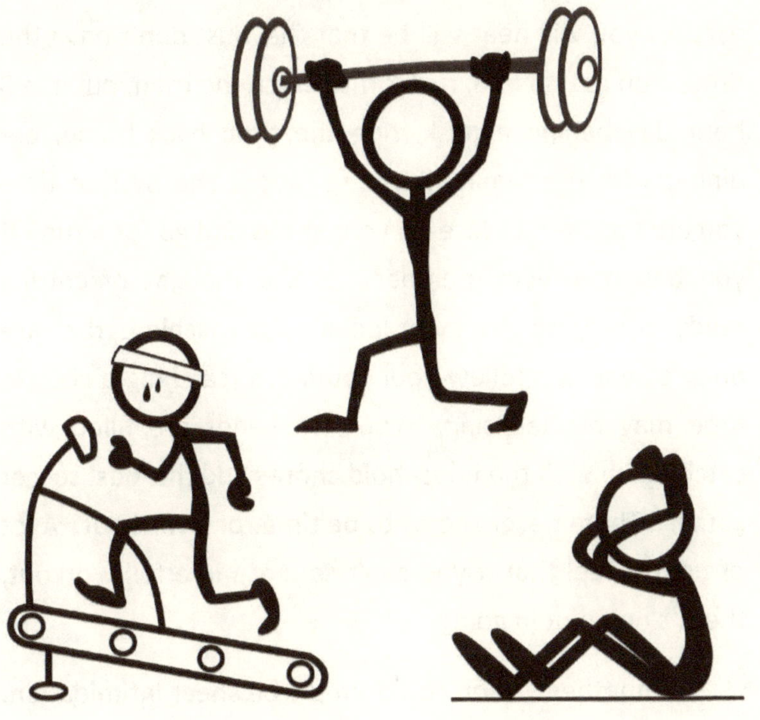

About Exercise (20% of focus)

About Exercise

There are many reasons that people have a hard time committing to an exercise program. One of the first excuses you will hear will be that they just don't have the time. You get up at 6, rush off to catch the train, put in a 8 hour day behind a desk, ride the train back home, eat dinner with the family (if you're lucky), and by that time you are too tired to lace up your shoes and go for a run. If you bought a gym membership, the thought of getting ready, driving to the gym, looking for machines that are open so you can follow your routine or catching a class in time may be daunting. Your weekends are filled with catching up with the household chores and the kids' soccer games. There never seems to be time for a workout. A lot of people feel that if you can't squeeze in a full workout, there's no point in going.

Another reason could simply be sheer intimidation. Ever walked into your local CrossFit gym in the middle of a workout? A bunch of people sweating to some loud music and all the clanking of barbells or medicine balls being slammed into the floor might be a little bit of sensory overload if it's been awhile since you've been in a gym! Even just going to a regular gym can be overwhelming.

Between the wide selection of machines that you have no idea how to use or trying to squeeze in a set next to a muscle bound meathead, waiting your turn to use a machine (or watching someone drip sweat all over the machine that you were planning on using), or trying to decide on how much weight to use can make it hard to get motivated. Maybe you want to try a Yoga or Pilates class. After seeing all of the regulars seamlessly going through the poses while you struggle to get into downward dog can make you feel like it's hopeless.

Another reason might be your current state of fitness. Maybe you're embarrassed about how you look in your workout clothes compared to others in the gym. If you have Instagram you can see many fitness accounts that will show off some pretty remarkable physiques. There's even fitness models that just show pictures of their butts in various locations. (Or so I've been told. I haven't actually seen any of them.) That can be very demotivating if you are comparing yourself to them. If you have tried before to get into shape and failed to hit your goal, you may have a mental block that tells you that you are just doomed to always be out of shape. Maybe you have had an injury or some general aches and pains and you're waiting for them to miraculously go away before you start a fitness program. Many people get injured when they start a new program by going at it too hard in the beginning. I know a couple of guys who get motivated to get back in shape once or twice a year and then hit the weights hard for two hours a day for a week straight. By the end of the first week, they are so sore they can barely move. Then, they have to take a week off just to recover. After a month with no gains, they stop going and the cycle starts all over again. It could also be the cost. Gym memberships aren't cheap. Most people can't afford a personal trainer to push them through every workout. Individual classes can also be pretty pricey. $15 for a yoga class may not seem that bad, but try going three times a week. On top of that, everything else has to fall into place for you to make it on a regular basis. If you can't get to the gym, you feel like you are wasting your money.

Here's some good news. None of these things are absolutely necessary for getting into and staying in shape. Now realize, I'm not trying to discourage you from any of the above. They are all great ways to get into shape. (Except maybe CrossFit. I don't know anyone who does CrossFit who isn't injured on a regular basis. I'm not hating on CrossFit, but it's too intense for the average person who just wants to get in good shape. Plus I'm jealous that my body is way too beat up to do it.) Buying a gym membership can be a great way to get motivated to start. Many gyms will also have reasonable rates on classes, if you buy in bulk. You can also get a personal trainer for 1-2 sessions just to show you how to use the machines and get a basic workout routine. Classes like

Zumba or Jazzercise can be fun ways to get a workout without having to come up with your own routine. It's also a good way to hang out with your friends while you exercise. My daughter is away at college and she and her friends look forward to going to Zumba to decompress after a long day of classes. None of these options will help though if you truly don't have the time or money to make it work.

That's why my personal approach to fitness has changed over the years. I have all of these excuses! First of all, I work in sales. Salespeople's schedules are a little more unpredictable than most because you have to be available around the client's schedule. Most of your clients don't come to you, so you spend a lot of time sitting in your car. I can't commit to being at the gym if I have the possibility of going to make money. Second, I'm not really intimidated of the gym simply because I've been working out for a long time. However, I do get grossed out at the thought of laying down on a bench or mat that numerous people have sweated on over the course of the day. As far as injuries go, don't get me started! In the last ten years, I've had a total knee replacement, (the other knee needs to be replaced at some point), torn rotator cuff surgery (by far the worst), and a partial wrist fusion. I also have two partially herniated discs in my back, bursitis in my elbow, and various other aches and pains from 17 years of working construction. I set off the metal detectors everywhere I go! I'm not using my injuries as excuse though. I'm using it as motivation for you. If I can be in good shape and still work out on a regular basis, anyone can. With my lack of flexibility due to metal in my body that doesn't move like regular joints, I couldn't keep up in a traditional yoga class to save my life. My best bet would be one of the classes in the pool you see the really old people doing. I'm not ready to take that step yet!

Here's the point. I don't do CrossFit. I don't have hour-long cardio sessions. I haven't done a bench press in 15 years. I would look really silly in a Zumba class. Yet I've maintained the same weight give or take 5 lbs. for the last 5 years. I have good muscle size and tone (people think I'm 10-15 lbs. heavier than I am due to my frame). I'm pretty flexible. So what do I do to achieve this? I go for walks. I do 10-20 minute cardio sessions at most. Most of my cardio is 5-10 minutes on my elliptical to warm up before I do my morning stretching routine which I will share with you. Most of my strength workouts are mini-workouts that I can do throughout the day in 5-10 minute bursts. I do body weight squats in a doorframe and calf raises on my steps for my legs. I do pushups on an incline on my stairs to take the strain off of my wrist and shoulder. I do pullups on my Total Gym which makes the load less on my joints. The most weight I use is a 15 pound dumbbell. I never do isolation exercises. Everything I do is geared toward working as many muscles as possible in as short of a time frame as possible as many times as I can manage. I try to make my life a workout. Some of the people who are in the best shape never work out at all. Look at your average construction worker or farmer. Their strength doesn't come from them doing curls or bench presses. It comes from swinging a hammer, carrying lumber, or pushing a wheelbarrow. Our ancestors were either walking to get to where the food and water was or they were actively hunting and carrying their food back to their family. They weren't doing burpees!

The main takeaway from this is that you need to use all of the reasons you're not exercising and then turn them around into reasons why you should exercise. If you're not exercising because you're too stiff, guess what? You need to start stretching! If you are embarrassed by the way you look, the only way to not be embarrassed is to get started on a program of health. You can use your bodyweight and your surroundings to do a majority of your workouts. If you want to make a dedicated area in your house a workout area, you will have a mini-gym that when you're rushed for time you can squeeze in a 10-30 minute workout that will leave you feeling better than when you started. I have a small 12'x12' section of my basement that is dedicated to my workouts. Almost all of my equipment I got used online. You'd be surprised how many people buy a machine, use it for two weeks, then never use it again (maybe you're one of them!). I also keep a 5 pound and 10 pound dumbbell in my office at work. Squeezing in a 5 minute workout is needed if I've been sitting at my desk for too long.

I won't lie. I used to be one of those guys who would be laughing when I heard that someone considered walking as a form of exercise. I agreed with all of the meatheads that if you weren't sweating like a pig at the end of your workout or if you weren't sore the next day you couldn't call it a workout. I would run for 30-40 minutes on an elliptical machine and congratulate myself on how many calories I had burned. The problem was for two days after that my knees were killing me and I had the same problem with my joints after a heavy lifting session. I changed my philosophy after I read the book "**The Primal Blueprint" by Mark Sisson**. I learned that your body is geared more towards walking for long periods of time with short bursts of intense exercise. The average hunter would track an animal for miles before engaging in a life or death struggle to get meat to bring back to his family. A gatherer may have to walk long distances to forage for berries or water and might make numerous trips in a day to keep her family fed and have a fresh supply of water. They rarely ran long distances. They didn't do long repetitious sessions of heavy lifting. This also ties in with the diet section. You might not eat all day long, then have a feast in the evening. I started incorporating this into my daily routine.

I try to go for a walk at least once a day, and more if I can find the time. Sometimes that might entail a long walk in the morning, a short walk mid-day, and another decent length walk in the evening, depending on the time of year. I have two black labs. They will walk for as long as I will take them! Having dogs will help force you to go for walks. It's just as good for them as it is for you. If you don't have a dog, what the hell is wrong with you? Dogs are awesome training partners!   You will never grab the leash and ask if they want to go for a walk only to have them say "No thanks!" They are always ready to go. I usually also listen to a podcast as we go for our morning walk. I listen to the Joe Rogan Experience daily. He has a wide variety of guests and the joy of listening to a podcast is that it's like being in the room with some very intelligent people while they are having an in-depth conversation. It's a great start to the day, not only for your body, but also your mind. According to Google, there are over 250,000 podcasts available. Surely, you can find one that will interest you. Start your day with some mental stimulation and it should benefit you for the rest of the day. Maybe you just prefer the calm of going for a walk first thing in the morning and listening to the birds chirping. Many of the things I wrote in this book came to me while I was on a walk. My mid-day walk might only be 10 minutes. Instead of a big meal at lunch, I might have a handful of almonds and an apple. I will then walk to the end of the street and back where my office is located. Do I get strange looks sometimes walking up and down the street in a dress shirt and slacks? Probably, but who cares? I'm doing this for myself. I've already gotten pretty used to getting strange looks from all of the other things I do to stay in shape.

Since you are going to use walking as exercise, it's extremely important that you walk correctly. A majority of people have lazy walking habits due to poor posture, tight muscles, and shoes that are heavily padded and doing most of the work for you. Some people have to use arch supports because their foot muscles are too weak. I'm a firm believer in minimalist or barefoot shoes with flat soles. There are a lot more muscles in your feet than you probably realize. Go get a foot massage and tell them to really work your arches and toes. The first time I did this, it sounded like someone squeezing a roll of bubble wrap. Most of the running shoes out there are heavily padded, especially in the heel. This points your foot down into a bad position similar to wearing heels or dress shoes. It also trains you to land on your heels and bounce back up instead of rolling through your foot and pushing off with the front of your foot. There's a reason that there is an expression regarding having a spring in your step. That's how your foot is supposed to operate. It also takes a lot of the strain off of your knees and lower back when you walk this way. The front part of your foot is acting as a shock absorber. You can find barefoot shoes on Amazon for relatively cheap. I have worn the Five Finger shoes from Vibram for many years. These shoes are great for teaching you the proper way to spread your toes the way nature intended. If you wear dress shoes or heels to work, you are pinching your toes together. Your toes are supposed to spread out for balance and leverage similar to how you would push something with your hands with your fingers spread out. If you try these shoes, go slowly until you get used to them. It took me about a month just to get used to putting these shoes on. **Do not** try running in these shoes until you have been wearing them on a regular basis. Even then you should only use them on softer surfaces, because there is no padding in these shoes. Concrete is not your friend. I recently bought a pair of QANSI barefoot shoes on Amazon for $35. I like the fact that they don't go in between each toe but have a wide toe area so you can spread your toes out. They also have slightly more padding and a little more arch support than the Five Fingers version and they are way less money (Can someone say endorsement opportunity?). I also like to wear Cole Haan dress shoes. They have a line of dress shoes with no heels. They feel like you are wearing running shoes.

Use your time walking as way to practice your perfect posture and technique. Everything that you do is based on muscle memory. Go try this experiment. Stand sideways in front of a full length mirror (No peeking!). Now stand as straight up as you can and lean back just a little so it feels exaggerated. Now take a look in the mirror. Chances are you are actually standing upright. Our bodies are so used to slouching forward from so many years of sitting at a computer, driving, and laying on your couch watching Netflix that standing up straight can actually start to feel unnatural. You have to practice bringing your body back in alignment to the way it used to be. Remember the image of the little old lady who is hunched over her walker? She didn't get that way over night. That was the result of too many years of gradual slouching. Her posture is literally pulling her forward.

I'm going to introduce a pose that I will refer to as perfect posture from here on out. Take off your shoes. Stand up straight. Try to spread your toes out as if you were trying to grip the earth to keep from falling off. The outside of your feet should line up with the outside of your hips. Your legs should be both lightly flexed and slightly bent at the knees. Gently tighten your stomach and push out your chest. Your shoulders should be pulled back with a tall neck and eyes straight ahead. This is perfect posture which will also be the position that you will start most of the exercises you will be learning. You will now step forward with your right foot and left arm swinging in tandem, big toe pointing forward. You should land on your heel but immediately roll forward onto the ball of your foot. Concentrate on spreading your toes and pushing off with the front of your foot. This should all be a fluid motion. Focus on maintaining your posture. Picture yourself walking down the catwalk. There should literally be a bounce in your step. Do this **every** time you go for a walk. You are training yourself to walk the way you are supposed to. If after a while you want to add a challenge, feel free to walk with a very light set of dumbbells. You can also do various exercises as you walk to get a better workout in. Make sure your focus is on your posture. You will have plenty of more opportunities to work your muscles! You should also focus on your breathing. Most people don't know how to breathe properly. It takes practice. You should be taking deep breathes that expand your stomach as well as your lungs. Breathe in deeply through your nose for a count of 5-6 feeling your chest expand then finishing in your stomach. Now breathe out deeply for a count of 6-7, starting with your stomach and then your lungs. Concentrate on your breath as you walk as well as your posture. Try not to get discouraged though when your mind wanders and you realize you're walking slouched or not breathing properly. It takes time to change bad habits. It won't happen all at once.

My next focus in exercise is the way my body operates. One of my main reasons for being in shape is to be able to continue to do things in my seventies that I can do now. Don't get me wrong. I hope that I'm in the position financially to be able to pay someone to take care of my lawn, rake my leaves, and paint my house as I get older so I can go out and do other fun things instead. I want to still be physically capable of doing them though. I have a mobility/flexibility routine that I do every morning and sometimes in the evening as well. Please don't confuse flexibility with mobility. Most people's idea of flexibility means holding a stretch for 30 seconds. This has no real life application though. You need to be flexible based on your muscles actually getting themselves into a certain position, not based on you pulling yourself into that position. I also do exercises for balance as well. You need to have an awareness of your body. Practicing balance now will save you from that fall later on in life. Make sure to have balance in your workouts as well. For every pushing exercise, do a pulling exercise. If you are doing some of the alternating arm exercises, start with your weak side first so you are strengthening both sides the same amount. If you do an exercise for your stomach, make sure to do one for your lower back. Alternate between an upper body and lower body exercise. This helps to maintain as close to a perfect symmetry as possible. The first thing most people need though is to loosen up their tight muscles and start to gain functionality. Here is my daily morning routine. This 10-15 minute routine done every day will help you live a more pain-free life.

First, I usually like to start off with a couple minutes of full body foam rolling. The older you get the tighter your muscles get. When you have tight muscles, you are more likely to do your exercises wrong or have bad posture. If you are consistently performing these exercises incorrectly you will develop bad form that will get worse as time goes on. Rolling around on a foam roller will start to loosen up your muscles. Most foam rollers will come with a DVD or some instructions with a routine on how to use it. I also use my foam roller before bed to help get a better night sleep. After you are loosened up, you are ready to begin the routine. Pay attention to how every exercise incorporates multiple body parts. This will help you to train your body to activate all of your muscles whenever you move. Start each of these movements by getting yourself into perfect posture when standing. Do 10-20 reps on each exercise, whatever feels best. Gradually increase the amount of reps when you start to feel stronger. I have also included illustrations to demonstrate most of these exercises. I have three basic workouts that I do on a regular basis, depending on how I feel, how much time I have to spare, and where I am. I try to do this morning routine daily.

Arm circles with high alternating knees. Get into perfect posture. Hold your arms out straight and do slow circles while alternating knee lifts. Go slow and make sure to really concentrate on maintaining perfect posture. Do 10-

20 arm circles in both directions. You can also slowly rotate in a circle while doing this exercise if you want to add in a balancing component.

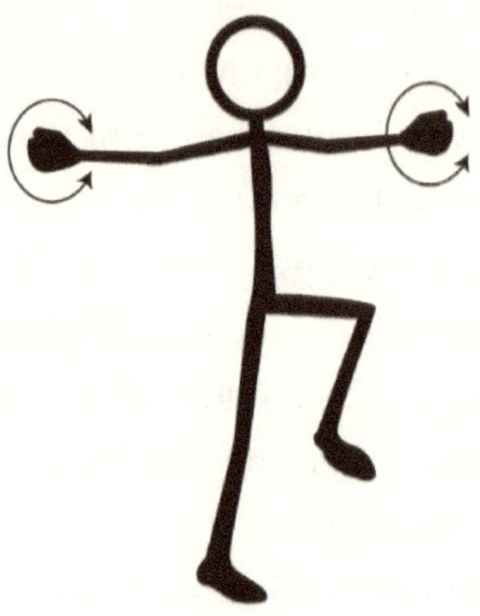

Shoulder stretch with band and calf raises. Start with your hands out in front of you shoulder-width apart gripping an exercise band. Pick a band that will make this easy. Remember, this is not a strength exercise. Have your feet shoulder-width apart with your toes pointing slightly out. Pull the band out until your arms are straight out in a perfect line and raise up on your calves. Raise up and pull at the same speed. If you start getting off balance you are going too fast. To get a different kind of stretch, you can also so this with your toes pointing in. On your last rep, hold the band straight out while maintaining perfect posture for 10-20 seconds. If your arms start to shake, you're holding it for too long.

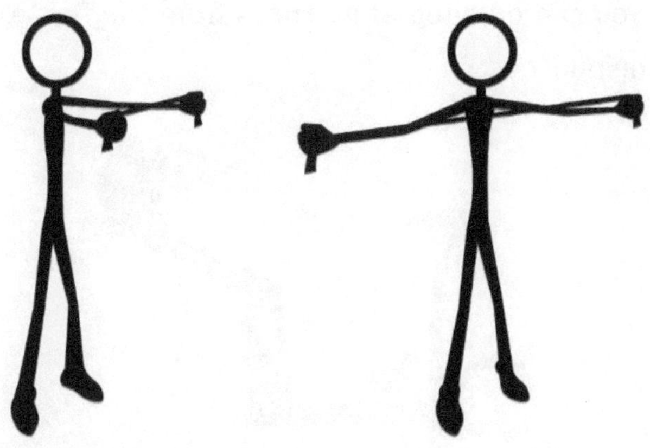

Fixed ½ crunch with dumbbell punches.   Lay on your back in the crunch position. Crunches are terrible for you because you are pulling your head towards your knees which teaches you bad posture. Instead, lay back in crunch position, pushing the small of your back down into the mat with your hands straight up in the air holding light dumbbells. Keep your head flat on the mat. I personally only use 5-8 pound dumbbells. You can also modify this exercise depending on your level of fitness. If this starts to hurt your back, put your feet straight up in the air while keeping your lower back tight to the floor. If the crunch position feels too easy, straighten your legs out to a 45 degree angle that is similar to the one hundred position in Pilates. Hold this position for as long as you possibly can without straining your back while you slowly throw alternating punches and squeeze the weights as if you're trying to crush them. If you want to take it to the next level, you can do alternating knees from the first exercise with the punches.

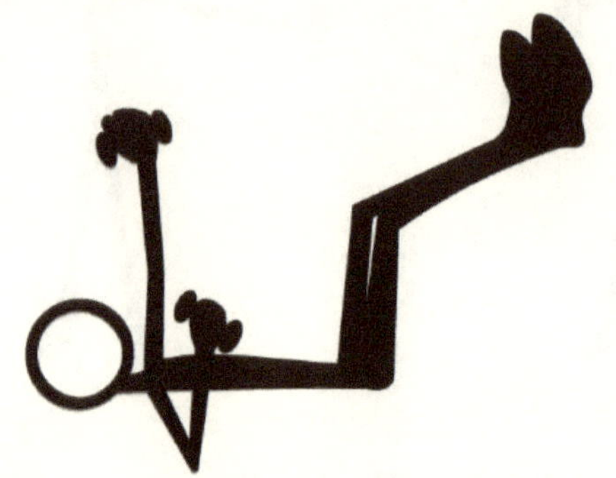

Hip raises with dumbbell flyes. Lay flat on your back with your knees bent and feet towards your butt. Your arms should be touching the ground with the back of your hands facing down. Slowly raise your hips and arms until you are in a straight line from knees to shoulder and your hands are touching directly over the center of your chest.

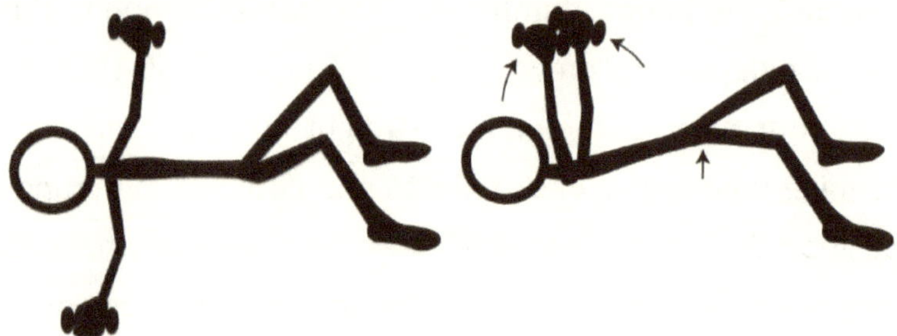

Rolling like a ball. This exercise is straight from Pilates. Lay on your back with your knees to your chest and hands wrapped around your shins. Sit up until your feet are an inch off of the ground. Roll back to starting position. It's important you do this slowly using your muscles to roll, not momentum. Eventually, you can get to the point where you can straighten out your legs and touch your toes to the ground behind your head. Work up to this position gradually. You don't want to hurt yourself!

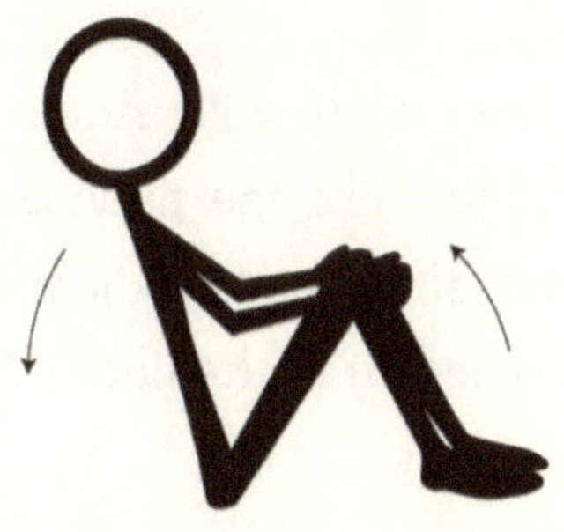

Alternate hamstring stretch. Lay on your back. Lift one leg up and reach forward slightly to grab your ankle. You are trying to stretch with your leg muscle, not by pulling your leg. Give your leg a slight pull (only an inch or two at most) then lower your leg and raise the other leg in a fluid motion.

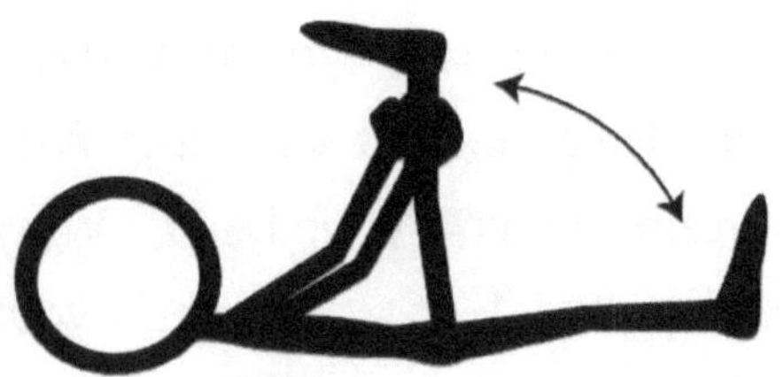

Swimming. Roll over on to your stomach. Stretch your arms and legs out just like the previous exercise. Take your right hand and left leg and lift them at the same time, only a couple of inches off of the floor. Go back and forth as if you were swimming.

Cat stretch. Come up on your hands and knees, looking straight ahead. Go back and forth between arching your back and pulling your pelvis down.

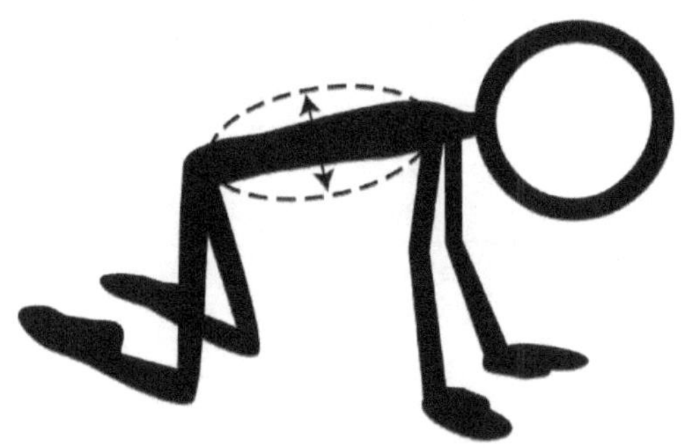

Alternate arm and leg stretch. Same starting position as Cat stretch. This time straighten your left arm and your right leg and hold for 5 seconds each time for a total of 10 for each side.

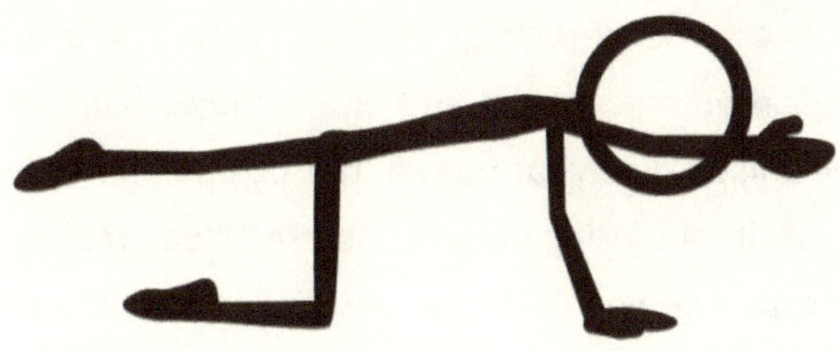

Fire hydrant. If you grew up in the eighties you might remember this exercise being the butt (pun definitely intended) of jokes. This is actually a great exercise to tighten your glutes but even more important it's great for loosening up those tight hips. Start in the cat stretch position only you're going to lift your leg up as if you were a dog peeing on a fire hydrant. Do this exercise slowly while really focusing on using your hip muscles, not using your momentum.

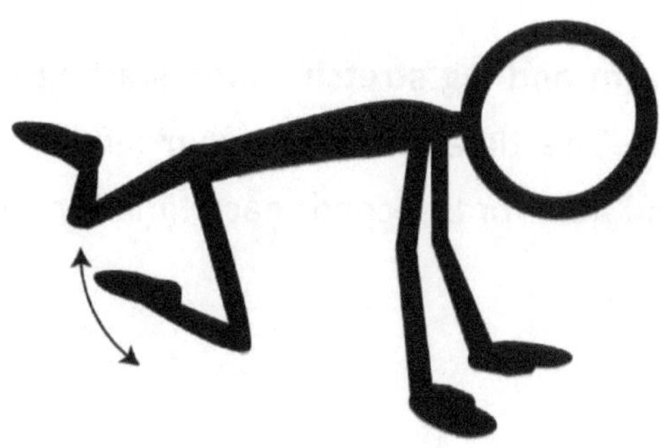

Plank.   Assume a pushup position except you will be resting on your forearms and your elbows bent at a 90 degree angle. Hold your body in this position for as long as you can without losing perfect posture. If you feel yourself starting to sag, you're done. Also, try to contract every muscle in your body as you hold this pose.   It will drastically shorten the amount of time you can do this. When you become advanced, you can do knee raises to the side while holding the plank.

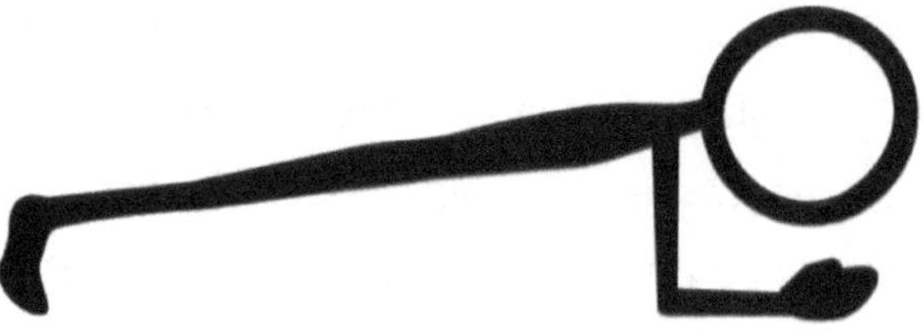

Cobra stretch.   You can Google the next 3 yoga poses if you aren't already familiar with them. These 3 poses are typically part of a sequence. Place your hips on the ground in plank pose and **gently** try to straighten your arms and stretch your back upwards. Do this 3-5 times slowly.

Child's pose. Get in the cat stretch position. Push your butt back on to your heels with your hands straight out in front of you. Try to lean back with your hips while stretching your arms out in front of you. Hold for 5-10 seconds and repeat a couple of times.

Downward dog with twist. Same position as child's pose except your legs are going to be straight, making your body form a triangle with the ground. Reach fully through your legs and arms and try to lengthen your body. After holding for 5 to 10 seconds, lift your left leg so that you have a straight line from your foot to your hands. Lightly twist your left leg to the right side of your body and look under your left armpit. Hold for 3- 5 seconds, then do the other side.

Finishing sequence. Stay in the downward dog position. Slowly walk your hands back until you can grab the back of your ankles. Take your hands and slide them up your legs as you straighten out. Take your hands up over your head and reach for the ceiling. Let your hands swoop out to the side as you do a slight back bend. Let them hang for 3-5 seconds then stand back up straight into perfect posture. Clinch all of your muscles and hold for 5-10 seconds. You're finished!

You should be feeling great when you are done. If you have time to squeeze in ten minutes of light cardio before you start this program it will help with the warmup but that's not necessary. I will also do this as a warmup before a strength workout, but it's great as a stand-alone workout. If you start every day with a brief workout you will start to notice that you are feeling more limber. After you've mastered the moves, feel free to switch the sequence around so you don't get bored.

The next workout will be my basic strength workout. This consists of only 5 exercises which will work every muscle in your body. This workout is strictly about gaining functional strength, not bulk. If you are a man, you will start to see small gains in size as you progress in reps. Most women will see a difference in muscle tone, but you shouldn't really gain much size due to the smaller amount of testosterone you produce compared to a man. All of the exercises are designed to use as many muscles as possible and also be as joint-friendly as possible. It's the same goal as the previous workout. You should feel better when you're finished. There's a huge difference between muscle soreness and having joint pain. You can push through soreness. Pain is an indicator that something might be wrong and that you should stop doing this exercise or modify it until there's no pain. The old school thinking of "No pain, No gain" doesn't apply to these workouts. You're training to gain functional strength, not to become Mr. (or Ms.) Universe! The first time you do this routine, you should try to do each of the exercises until you can't do it anymore without maintaining your form. Write those numbers down and on your next workout do 2-3 reps less than that number. Do this workout 2-3 times a week and add a rep or two every week. After a month, go for your max again. You should be pleasantly surprised with your gains. If you try to only add just 1 rep every single week, you could potentially add anywhere between 30-50 reps by the end of the first year. Now that's pretty impressive! Here's your list of the 5 strength exercises. You should already know how to do these exercises.

Pushups. This is probably the single best exercise you can do in terms of working your entire body. Now maybe it's been a while since you've done a pushup. If so, you want to start out slowly. You need to perfect your form before you start trying to crank out some regular pushups. Stand in perfect posture arms-length away from a wall. Put your arms out straight shoulder-width apart and hands flat against the wall. Slowly lower your body towards the wall while maintaining perfect posture. Your feet should be flexed and you should feel it in your ankles and calves as you move forward. Your legs, core and chest should be tight as well. Do this exercise slowly (2-3 seconds down, 2-3 seconds up) and concentrate on feeling all of your muscles contract as you do this. After you've done this to the point that you can complete 50 reps, you're ready for the next progression which is stair pushups. You can still start with this variation as a warmup before moving on to the stairs. It's the same sequence only you're doing it on an angle. I do these at work throughout the day on the railing at my office. You can also use a desk or table as long as it's stable. It will be a little painful, plus slightly embarrassing to face plant on your desk because it moved in the middle of a pushup! I never do regular pushups due to my wrist fusion, but if you've mastered the angle pushup feel free to go for it. Just be sure you are still maintaining a straight line from your heels to shoulders. If your back starts to sag, you are doing more damage than good at that point and you should stop.

Pullups. I don't ever do traditional pullups anymore due to my joint issues. If you can, great! If not, I highly recommend getting a Total gym. You can get one used between $100- $300 depending on how much you want to spend. (Unless Total Gym wants me to be their new spokesperson when Chuck Norris retires. Then you should totally buy a new one!) I have the most basic model. You can do many exercises on it, but my favorite is an incline pullups. Doing an incline pullup takes some of the strain off of your joints, and if you're not strong enough yet to lift your body weight with a traditional pullup, you can lower the angle to make it easier. I like to do around 20-30 reps for a nice burn with no pain afterwards. Do this exercise slowly as well. Make sure your shoulders are in line and squeeze the bar as tightly as possible. When you are pulling yourself up, visualize that you are squeezing a tennis ball between your shoulder blades. This way you won't be using just your arms. If you don't buy a Total gym, you can get pullup bars that fit in your doorway or you can also take an exercise band and put it over an open door and kneel in front of the door to mimic the pullup motion. Just make sure to use a light tension exercise band and do slow reps. The last thing you want is to use a heavy band and pull your door out of whack!

Dumbbell military press with alternating arm and leg/calf raises. Stand in perfect posture with a light dumbbell in each in hand with your arms parallel to the floor and your elbows bent up at a 90 degree angle. If you have a low ceiling you can also do this on your knees, just make sure your torso is straight. The heaviest weight I use for this exercise is 15 pounds. Slowly raise your right arm and bring your left knee up at the same time. After you've alternated back and forth to the point where you feel your form going, stop and get back into the starting position. Now, you're going to lift both arms at the same time and simultaneously raise up on your toes activating your calf muscles for a few reps. Go slowly so you don't lose your balance.

Squats. Many people don't like to do squats because it hurts their back or knees. Usually it's because they are using poor form or they are using too much weight. The best way to eliminate that problem is to do body weight squats holding onto a doorway or a post. I do my squats in my basement holding onto a support column. Stand in a doorway or next to a support column with your body a couple of inches away. Place your hands flat on the sides of the doorway to balance, not to pull yourself up. Put your nose a couple of inches away and keep your nose the same distance away as you begin to lower yourself to the floor. Go slowly and really concentrate on feeling it in your lower back, glutes, quadriceps, and calf muscles. Only go down to the point that you feel a good stretch. As you do your reps you will start to naturally go lower as your muscles loosen up. Go down until it starts to get difficult and then don't go any lower. Really focus on the muscles that you are activating. Remember that your goal is to feel better and looser after this exercise, not in pain. After you've mastered this form of squat, you can move on to a goblet squat. Stand away from the door with a dumbbell in your hands, pushed up under your chin. Try to go down in the same motion as you did in the doorway. I like to do some doorway squats before I do a goblet squat just to dial in my form.

Plank. Time for the grand finale! Now that you've activated every muscle in your body, drop down into the plank position that you learned in the first workout. Tighten all of those muscles you've been using and hold until you feel you're starting to lose your form. Push your body up to downward dog and complete the entire finishing sequence from the previous workout. That's it!

This workout should leave you feeling slightly tired, but in a good way. If you do the warmup routine, then after you're done with this workout you should feel really good. You should **never** feel pain during this workout. If you do, stop that particular exercise and reposition your hands or move on to a different exercise. After you've mastered this workout, feel free to change it up a bit by doing different speeds of reps. Some days you can go nice and slow. Some days you can speed it up and try to do more reps. Just make sure that your form doesn't suffer. You can also do a version where you lower slowly but come up faster. This is good for developing your fast-twitch muscles. The nice thing about this workout is you won't need to warm up first if you don't have time. You will gradually warm up as you start the exercises.

There are multiple variations to the exercises I've listed. As you become more fit, you can mix things up. Side planks work a whole different group of muscles than a traditional plank. Moving your hand position changes the areas that you are targeting when you're doing pushups. If you are performing a chin up (palms facing you) instead of a traditional pullup (palms facing away) you will be using your biceps muscles more and your back and shoulder muscles less. Try to change things up. It will keep you from being bored.

My other workout is usually a Pilates or Yoga video. There are many of these online that you can watch for free. You can also get them at your local library. Experiment with a lot of different videos and if you find a few that you really like, go buy them online. The benefit to doing the same exercises in the same order each time allows you to learn the poses and sequences to the point that you don't have to watch the video, you can just listen. This will give you a nice flow as you transition between poses. I like to do this once or twice a week just to change things up. Most videos have different levels based on your experience level, so you can work up to harder workouts as you get more proficient at the poses. I personally like the DDP Yoga program from former professional wrestler Diamond Dallas Page. His program is his own combination of yoga, isometrics, and strength training. I highly recommend it if you have joint issues. I usually only do one cardio workout a week. I have an elliptical machine that I will run on for 25-30 minutes just to work up a nice sweat. If you use an elliptical, don't use the arm part. This will help to work on your balance as well as get your heart pumping. Please start out at a slow speed until you get the hang of it. You don't want to wipe out and get hurt!

Before I had my knee replacement done I had a NordicTrack ski machine. This was by far my favorite machine for cardio. Using the hand part was much more natural than an elliptical, and it is way harder physically. The first time I tried it, I barely made it for a full 10 minutes! I don't recommend jogging until you are already in good shape. The excess weight will make it harder on your joints, especially your knees, ankles, and hips. Wait until you've dropped the weight and try to run on grass if you can. Walk, then run. I also don't recommend an exercise bike. If you're trying for functional fitness, it's better to be running than sitting. However, if you enjoy biking outdoors, go for it. I used to like to go for long rides on a local bike path through the woods before my knees started to hurt too much. There's a Zen-like feeling you get on long bike rides away from civilization. The best exercise is the one that you enjoy.

In terms of equipment necessary for a home gym, the list is brief. You will need one piece of equipment for cardio. If you have a low ceiling that limits you from getting an elliptical or NordicTrack (I personally have to take out a ceiling tile to do mine), get a rowing machine or a HealthRider instead of an exercise bike. This will at least work out your upper body as well as your lower body. Next, you'll need a few dumbbells. These allow you to do alternating lifts with your opposite leg for strength and balance. Start with small weights. This is going to help you to learn proper form and also help with your balance. Once you have the form down, you can always use heavier weights. I also use an array of exercise bands. The exercise bands are fantastic for hitting different ranges of motion. When you do a dumbbell press, it's hardest when the weight is closest to you and easiest when your arm is straight. With bands, it's the opposite. It gets harder as you tighten the band. If you can find a setup that attaches to a door even better. Sometimes I'll go down in my basement and throw as many punches as I can then turning around and doing a series of pulls. Individual bands are also great for the office or if you're going to travel. Throw them in the suitcase and pull them out for a 10-15 minute workout as soon as you get to your hotel. I also have a padded yoga mat for my floor routine. As I've said before, I highly recommend getting a Total Gym. You can do over 50 modified exercises on this machine and you can even use it as a reformer for Pilates. You say you want to get in some cardio but you only have 5 minutes? Go buy a jump rope. 5 minutes of intense rope jumping will be better for your fitness than a boring jog around a track. I also use a wobble board for balance and to help with strengthening my ankles. Rolling a golf ball along the bottom of your foot to break up tension then jumping on the wobble board is a great way to start any workout. If you want a 2 minute total body workout, grab a set of light dumbbells. As you begin rotating the board in a circle, do some alternating curls. Be sure to take your arm that's coming back and extend it behind you to activate your triceps (the muscle on the back of your arm) to get a nice push/pull workout. If you are in perfect posture, you are now working almost every single muscle in your body. It's also great for balance and the smaller stabilizer muscles you won't activate with traditional exercises. After you've gone around one full rotation, go back in the other direction and also change the position of your hands. Do one rotation with your palm up, the next with palm facing vertically. This will help activate the different parts of your forearm, biceps, and triceps. Another component for balance and stabilizer strength is a Swiss ball. You can do a lot of exercises on a Swiss ball that feel very different than doing them on a bench. There are many exercise books that are specific to the Swiss ball. After you have mastered the routines that I've laid out, get a Swiss ball and take it to the next level.

Last, but definitely not least, would be getting exercise by doing something you love to do. Go join a softball league. See if your local park district offers tennis lessons. Go take a martial arts class. Get your girlfriends to commit to going to Zumba a couple times a week. As I've said before, the best form of exercise is the one that you really enjoy and will stick with.

Most exercise programs will begin with a disclaimer about how you should see your doctor before beginning this plan. Since all of the exercises are very basic, I don't believe this is necessary (I should probably check with my legal team first), but I do highly recommend getting a deep tissue massage.   Find a massage therapist who also performs other forms of physical therapy. Schedule a 1-1½ hour long deep tissue massage and stretching session. I used to have horrible back pain. No matter what back exercises I did, I would have to go to the chiropractor at least once every 2-3 weeks to get adjusted. When I started going to my therapist (Shout out to Kristy Lancaster at Y-Knot Move!), I learned that a majority of my back problems had to do with tight hips, legs, and feet, as opposed to my back. Getting the deep tissue massage helped me to have an awareness of my muscles. She gave me specific exercises to loosen my hips that helped ease my back pain to the point that I only have to go in now every 2-3 months for general maintenance. She also turned me on to using a foam roller for general self-massage and a lacrosse ball if I had any specific areas that are tight. If you can find one who also does Functional Movement Screens, even better. This test will show you where your imbalances are, so you can work on fixing them. This will go a long way towards you feeling better and will also make sure that you are able to perform your workouts without doing any more damage due to muscle imbalance.

The next section will be me walking you through how to implement this into your own daily routine. I'll try to show you how you can incorporate all of these ideas into your own life. Remember, this isn't a get fit quick program. This is about you taking your busy life and then figuring out how to make it better. If you have a flexible plan for your week it will make it a lot easier for you to continue with your improving fitness. The more times that you successfully adapt to changes in your schedule the more it will start to just be part of who you are. Let's look at how to do that!

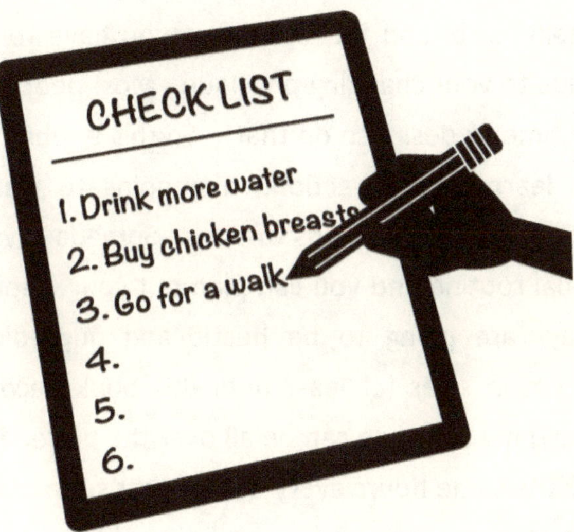

Putting it all together

Putting it all together

This is the part of the book where most fitness authors will lose you. After you've digested (pun intended) all the information on how to eat and exercise, they will give you a super-detailed workout with specific sets and reps to follow. Then you will have to do some crazy calculations to figure out your daily calorie intake and protein, carb, and fat ratios that you have to adjust weekly due to your changing physique. Most people don't have the time or desire to do that! So this is what you're going to learn in this section. I'm going to walk you through a few different kinds of days. Somedays you are in a normal routine and you can plan out your whole day. Some days are going to be hectic and unpredictable. Because I'm in sales (at least until this book becomes a best-seller!) my schedule can be all over the place. Maybe you work the same hours every day. If that's the case, you shouldn't have any excuse for not being able to come up with something that works for you. If you live a busy lifestyle (who doesn't?) then these tips will help you to integrate this into your busy schedule.

The first part will be dialing in your nutrition. One of the first things you learn in most books is you're supposed to go into your fridge and pantry and throw away all of the junk food. You go to the store and buy the exact grocery list that they provide and make all of your meals according to their recipes and eat at the times they specify. However, most of you probably have a spouse or children who will get pissed if you throw away their treats! You are doing this for yourself. Don't worry about changing anyone else's habits of eating until you have completely changed your own. Nobody likes having a diet plan forced on them. Try to make a grocery list that has as many healthy options as possible. Eliminating all of the bad food from your house won't be as helpful as you might think. If there's no bad food in the house it's easy to stay true to your plan. The first time you are faced with temptation however, it is very easy to go off the rails. By having some temptation and ignoring it, you will slowly start to reinforce good habits. That way when you're hungry and you have a choice between an apple and a handful of cookies, hopefully you'll pick the apple! Once again, you will fail occasionally on this plan. Sometimes when you fail it can actually help to strengthen your willpower. One of my favorite quotes about this comes from a man named Eugene Sandow. Sandow was a strong-man from back in the late 1800's. His quote is **"The man (or woman) who means to make his/her body as perfect as possible must cultivate habits of self-control and of temperance. The man (or woman) who has**

cultivated his/her body has also cultivated self-respect."
This is a journey of self-improvement, not perfection. Every time you are faced with a temptation and you don't succumb to it, you are now strengthening your resolve. If you stick to any kind of plan, whether it's a diet/exercise plan or some other self-improvement plan, you will start to feel better about yourself. I've been thinking about writing a book for a long time. Once I actually committed to it, I started to get excited which added fuel to the fire. Every day I made myself go down in my basement and sit down at my computer to write, I always felt better about myself afterwards. If you are having a hard time getting started with any type of self-improvement program, read the book **"The War of Art" by Steven Pressfield**. His book is about how people have this built-in resistance to changing and improvement. Sometimes the hardest thing is just to get started. Once momentum kicks in though it gets a lot easier. If you're trying to lose some weight, there's not too many things that are as gratifying as having to go out to buy a smaller size of clothes because your old clothes are too big or having someone you haven't seen in a while ask you if you have lost weight! Use that feeling to buy healthy foods and then actually eat them!

The next part after you have the food is what you do with it. I eat a lot of grilled chicken. To cook every day is impossible for me. I will cook 5-6 chicken breasts at a time so I will have them ready to cut up when I need it.

My daughter has now gotten into the habit of making salads to take to work simply because the chicken is readily available. I'm not going to tell you what exactly to eat because everybody's tastes are different and your schedule of eating is different as well. My schedule is usually different every day. Some days I will eat three meals if I know I'll have the time. I will start off the day with 4-5 scrambled eggs and an avocado on some days, some days I will have a protein shake. Protein shakes are one of your best friends if you have a busy schedule and don't have the time to make a complete meal. They are also great if you are trying fasting but you don't think you can make it all the way to lunch without eating. You can drink a shake at your desk. It's a great way to get nutrients from things that you might not normally eat. Mushrooms are good for you. However, I just can't handle the texture of mushrooms. There are a lot of options at your local health food store for organic dehydrated vegetable powders that you can add to a shake that won't really add too much flavor. My typical morning shake will have a combination of 16 ounces of water and unsweetened almond or coconut milk. I will then add a teaspoon of mushroom powder, a scoop of organic super greens powder, a scoop of either whey or plant protein powder, two tablespoons of ground flaxseed, a spoonful of peanut butter or almond butter, a tablespoon of coconut or olive oil, a big handful of spinach or kale, a few broccoli florets or cauliflower, and a ½-1 cup of frozen berries or a half of a banana. Add a couple of ice cubes and blend. You are getting an entire meal of health in a single glass. You may have to work up to this gradually. Start off at first with just the protein powder, peanut butter, and berries and slowly start adding other healthy things as you get used to the flavors. A word of caution: If you are not used to eating this healthy, make sure to have a bathroom nearby. This shake is like Drano for your intestines. You may need a bathroom break shortly after finishing! Another great way to get all of your nutrients in one meal is a salad like I described earlier. Adding some form or multiple forms of greens, broccoli, grape tomatoes, shredded carrots, shredded red cabbage, sunflower seeds, shaved almonds or walnuts, olive oil, avocados, pure cheese (not pre-shredded cheese that has chemicals in it to keep the cheese separated) and some form of meat (chicken, fish, steak, etc.,) along with a healthy dressing will give you a complete meal. Mix it up with different combinations and salad dressings. Go out and buy a couple of big containers so that you have something to throw this all together in and take it to work with you. There are many recipes online for healthy salad dressings. Most commercial dressings uses soybean oil or vegetable oil as a main ingredient. Avoid these types of dressing. It's like adding some poison to your healthy salad. I try to stick to something that uses Greek yogurt as a base. I will put

1-2 tablespoons of olive oil on first and mix up my salad before adding the salad dressing. Adding oil to your salad helps you to absorb the nutrients better and causes you to use less dressing.

If I'm fasting until lunch, I usually only eat two meals. I will also eat two large meals if I know it's going to be a busy day. I will have a large breakfast of healthy fats, fiber, and protein and that will usually keep me full until dinner. Take all of the principles about eating that you have learned and just incorporate them into two meals instead of three. There really is no difference between eating three normal size meals or two big meals as far as maintaining a healthy body composition. Having to eat three meals a day is something that was sold to us by food companies that want you to eat more food! Our ancestors probably only ate two meals a day if they were lucky. If you don't have time to eat enough vegetables and fruit, you can supplement with some organic super greens and water in a shaker cup. Drinking a cup of super greens and dehydrated mushrooms is as gross as you probably think it sounds. To make it even more disgusting, I will add a tablespoon of apple cider vinegar and a teaspoon of some form of fiber. Here's how I look at it. It only takes about 10 seconds to drink this miserable concoction, but the benefits are well worth it. If I add that to my eggs and avocado, I am having a complete meal. Don't feel bad if you are not able to eat a complete meal every single time.

Our ancestors ate whatever was available. One day they may have only had berries and seeds, the next day they might have had only meat. It won't harm you to skip one or the other occasionally. If the thought of not eating between breakfast and dinner is too daunting, you can also add a small snack between the two meals if necessary at first. At some point you shouldn't need the snacks. This is all part of the fasting process that your body will get used to over time.   I keep a box of 100- calorie almonds/walnuts mix in my car. If I don't have time to stop for lunch I'll eat a couple of these with a bottle of water. My hunger will go away then until I'm able to have a real meal. If I don't have time (or am just too lazy) to make something to bring for dinner I'll stop at Chipotle (Working on those sponsorships! Maybe I could be the new Chipotle guy. Kind of like Jared from Subway, without the high-profile arrest). A burrito bowl with beans, meat, salsa, and guacamole is a complete meal that will leave you satisfied for a long time. If you don't happen to have a Chipotle nearby, stop somewhere that has similar options. Take the principles that you have learned in this book and start incorporating them into your daily routines. If you need help with recipes, go online and use the countless resources of the internet to find healthy recipes. This is not a cook book. It's a philosophy book! You'll have to do some leg- work on your own. It really is as easy as I'm making it out to be. As I said before, the healthier you eat, the more you will start to crave not only healthy foods but the feeling you get after eating healthy foods. I do love the taste of pizza, but I hate the feeling of bloating I get after I've eaten it. I much rather have the lightness I feel in my belly after a big salad. Being full of healthy nutrients is different than being stuffed! I'm at the point where I don't really crave chips or pretzels anymore. I prefer some carrots or broccoli florets dipped in hummus. If you incorporate this knowledge into your own personal philosophy and try to follow the 85% rule it will be almost impossible to not start seeing immediate improvement. The other benefit to eating clean is that eventually you will get down to what would be considered your ideal weight. Your body knows what the right weight for you is based on your age, metabolism, and your general activity level. When I first started trying to lose weight, my goal was to get to 170 pounds. On my old program of focusing strictly on trying to lose weight I could just never get there. I would get down to 172-173, then I would fall off of the wagon for a day or two. Next time I checked I was back up to 175. Talk about an endless cycle of discouragement! As soon as I began to focus strictly on health, a funny thing started to happen. I breezed past 170 without really trying. Then, even with eating around the same amount of calories over the next few months I wound up getting down to 165 without adding any additional exercise. That seems to be my ideal weight. If you are planning on using a scale to track your progress, realize there are many factors that will affect your weight. My advice would be to only weigh yourself on Monday and Friday mornings. Do it first thing in the morning. That way you are getting the two extremes if you are following the plan of eating healthy during the week and then having reward meals during the weekend. Your weight can fluctuate as much as 4-5 pounds depending on what you ate and drank. You should get to the point of where you are around a pound less every Friday from the previous week. It might not seem like much, but just like your progression in strength if you were to lose a pound a week you could lose 30-50 pounds over the course of the year. That's pretty impressive! If you try to make a goal of losing 30-50 pounds, it might seem impossible. Shooting for a pound a week is achievable. Give yourself a small reward every 5 pounds. It will give you something to look forward to. Just focusing on diet will help. The best way to guarantee success though is to also exercise on a consistent basis.

I usually start off every day with the routine you learned about in the exercise section that will warm up your muscles and performing stretches that will get your blood pumping to start your day. This will only add 10- 15 minutes to your morning routine. You say you get up at 4:30 in the morning to catch the train? My response is get up at 4:15 then. Getting up that early sucks either way. 15 minutes earlier isn't going to make that big of a difference. At least you'll feel much better on the train. Plus, it's also great reinforcement for your new healthy lifestyle to start the day with a short workout.   My schedule does vary greatly depending on the time of year. There are times when we are slow that I will have the option of getting in a full workout in the morning. During those times I might do a strength workout one day. The next day might be Yoga or Pilates. The next day might be cardio. Sometimes I won't have that luxury though. When that is the case I then have to improvise and spread my workouts out over the course of the day. You can start to make exercising a habit that you can incorporate any time that you have 5-10 minutes to kill. When I get back to my office after an appointment, I usually come in the side door to my building that has a few steps and a landing with a railing. Before I go in, I will put my briefcase down, do a set of calf raises on the stairs, then go over to the railing and do a set of pushups. Other times I may go directly into my office and do a set of bodyweight squats in my doorway. Total time: 3 minutes. I will do the same routine whenever I go downstairs to my basement. Over the course of the day I might workout 5-10 times for 2-5 minutes at a time. This will add up over time. When I go out to cut my grass I have to pick up the dog poop and sticks, weed whack around the perimeter, and then cut the grass. This will require 2-3 trips to the garage. Every trip I grab my jump rope and do at least 100 revolutions. If

I'm working on a project and have to go back and forth to my basement, I will jump on my Total gym and crank out some pullups instead of the pushups. I might do one-legged calf raises instead of both legs at the same time. Sometimes I will point my toes in, sometimes out. I always park at the back of the parking lot at the grocery store. I try to always take the stairs instead of the escalator or elevator. I keep a variety of small dumbbells at my office. I was going to describe the workout as a separate office workout, but I would have been stealing the entire routine. Buy the book **"Super Body, Super Brain" by Michael Gonzalez-Wallace.** This book will show you how doing certain exercises will not only work your muscles but also help to stimulate your brain and central nervous system. It's also helpful for balance and will wake you up even better than a cup of coffee. I try to do this every day around 2-2:30 PM if I'm in my office. It has helped to eliminate my need for that afternoon jolt of caffeine. You will actually feel better after you do one of these mini-workouts. I keep a Gripmaster in my car to work on my hand strength when I'm driving. (Note from my legal team. Always keep both hands on the wheel in the 10 and 2 position just like you learned in Drivers Ed. Please be safe!) Grip strength is one of the first things to go as you get older. I want to be able to open my own jars in my old age!

Only you can know your routine and how you can incorporate this into your life. The point is you need to move if you want to be in the kind of shape you need to be in to have the kind of life you want to have. If you stop moving, you start dying, plain and simple. Make your life your workout. As I mentioned earlier, don't worry about the strange looks you might get. The people in my office are now used to seeing me doing pushups on the stair rail. I've gotten many strange looks from my neighbors when I'm out cooking burgers on the grill and started doing high alternating knees or calf raises with my toes pointed out to the side like a ballerina. You will feel self-conscious at first, but you'll get used to it. Become known as the fitness person. You may be surprised at how many people might start coming up to you and asking for help with their own fitness. That's a really rewarding feeling! Make this part of your new philosophy. Do these little additions to your routine every day. At some point, you'll do them without even thinking about it.

The last part is just a few tips on what to do if you would like to see rapid improvements in a short period of time. Most of these ideas are just expanding on what you have learned previously. The first tip is just to move faster! Skip the walks and spend some time doing longer periods of cardio in your fat burning state. To find your fat burning heart rate, you take your age and subtract it from 220 to find your maximum heart rate. Your fat burning rate will be 70% of your maximum heart rate. You can get a heart rate monitor on Amazon. When you work out at that rate, your body will burn fat for a few hours after you are done exercising, as long as you don't eat anything. I try to wait 1 hour after exercising before I eat anything. Your body is burning fat and is also producing growth hormone during that time. Once or twice a week you can add some interval sprinting at the end of your cardio. Take your last five minutes of your cardio and sprint at full speed for 10-15 seconds, then walk for 45-50 seconds. Do 4-5 sets, then walk for a few minutes to cool down. Doing this will really rev up your fat burning. You can also take the strength workout and do 2-3 circuits instead. Make sure to take a day in between these workouts to prevent joint issues or over-working your muscles. I will do my strength workout on Wednesday and Sunday to give myself time to recuperate. As far as diet goes, the best thing you can do for losing weight rapidly is to eliminate all carbs until you get down to the weight you want. I personally have had great results by doing a strict carnivore diet. That is exactly what it sound like. Nothing but meat! I will add avocado, eggs, and my super green powder to make sure I'm getting additional nutrients. This probably isn't the best diet for the long term, but it's extremely effective and should be safe for you to do short-term. It is also good to use as an elimination type diet. Many people eat food that they may have a hard time processing, even if they're not allergic to it. Try this for a couple of weeks then begin to slowly add some other foods back in. You may find that certain foods may cause you to feel bloated or constipated after you start eating them again. This will help you to find the right kind of foods for your body. Lastly, do a 24 hour fast at least once a week. Try to go from dinner to dinner to make it easier. As far as the tips go, this is really all that you will need. If you follow the concepts in this plan, you will get to where you're at your ideal weight. If you have any sudden weight gains due to a vacation or the holiday season, a couple of weeks of these tips will get you right back to where you want to be. I recently took part in a six week extreme physique challenge with some of my younger co-workers. I was getting bored with my workout routine and wanted to add a spark. The only things that I added to my routine was pushing harder on my strength and cardio workouts and also eliminating alcohol. I dropped five pounds in six weeks and actually had a six pack for the first time ever (It was gone within two days!). It really isn't that hard to get the kind of body you want.

This can be a life changing book if you will follow these principles. If you're lucky, it will not only change your life. You can also help create change in other people after they start to see the results from your hard work. I can't describe the satisfaction I've gotten over the years from helping other people to get started on the path to better health. The more that you spread your knowledge and experience, the more it will help you by reinforcing it in your own brain. The funny thing about writing this book is that there are things that I had stopped doing or had forgotten about until I started writing it down. I am still a work in progress. The best thing you can do for yourself is to continue learning about fitness. I will have a list of books and podcasts for you to help continue your journey. It's 2019. There have been many new breakthroughs in health, supplementation, and longevity in the past few years. Staying up to date with the latest information will help you to improve your health beyond the things you've learned in this book. It will also help you with positive reinforcement and staying motivated. I almost always notice a much higher level of intensity in both my exercise and my diet after listening to a good podcast or reading a good book about health. You can have a great life of health if you apply what you've learned in this book. There is always room for improvement though. Try to be the best you can be. It will only make your life better!

Make the commitment to yourself to just get started. Take baby steps at first and slowly begin to incorporate all of the things that you have read into your daily routine. Understand that you will fail occasionally and be okay with it. You can always get back on course. You owe it to yourself to give yourself the best chance at a long, healthy life. Get started now! I hope that you get as much out of reading this book as I did writing it. If so, share the book with a friend. They will thank you in the end. Good luck with your new healthy body!

James Shropshire

January 25, 2019

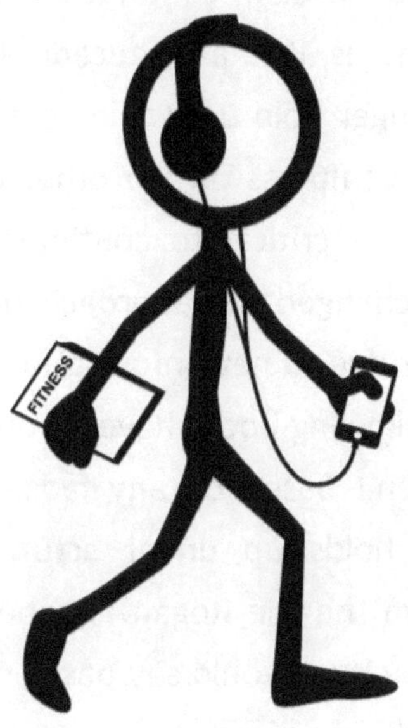

Recommended books and podcasts

Recommended reading and podcasts

I'm a big believer in continued learning. Many of the beliefs we had as little as a decade ago about health and fitness no longer hold up. I think continuing to learn, whether it is about fitness or any other type of personal development skill is critical to continuing to grow as a person. I have changed my approach on many things I used to hold dear due to new information (Fat-free yogurt anyone?). The following books have stood the test of time because they aren't based on any fads, but on timeless knowledge that holds up under scrutiny. All of the podcasts are from the Joe Rogan Experience. If you are offended by profanity, I would say pass on these, but they do hold a wealth of information and also will help to strengthen your own philosophy. Some of these guests are a bit extreme, but they are some of the more interesting podcasts. Remember, the more you get into a fitness lifestyle, the easier it is to maintain. Here are the books and podcasts that influenced this book the most.

Books:

"The Primal Blueprint" by Mark Sisson. I may be beating a dead horse here, but this is one of the most important books I've read as far as changing my perspective on how to eat as well as how often to exercise. If you are interested in a more scientific version of my book then this would be the best book for you to start.

"The New Evolution Diet" by Art DeVany. I actually read this book before "The Primal Blueprint." It is a very similar book, just written from a slightly different perspective. I believe it's good to read a couple of books that are similar because everyone has different learning styles. One book may resonate with you more than the other. It will also help to reinforce the concept of eating and exercising like our ancestors.

"The Four Hour Body" and "Tools of Titans" by Tim Ferriss. Both books are full of life hacks to help you get in better shape. TOT also has a lot of great interviews on pretty much every subject you might be interested for self-improvement.

"Man 2.0: Engineering the Alpha" by John Romaniello and Adam Bornstein. This is a great book for men (Sorry ladies. I don't have a specific book to recommend for you.) which explains how what you eat and when can affect your production of testosterone and growth hormone. It has an entire plan of eating and exercise to help you make a massive change in your physique in a relatively short amount of time

"Convict Conditioning" by Paul Wade. If you want to expand your strength workouts to develop your functional strength, this is the only book you will ever need. Body weight exercise strengthens your muscles and your joints. Wade shows you how to master the basics of each exercise and also walks you through the progressions to take it to the next level.

"Super Joints" by Pavel Tsatsouline. After you have mastered my morning routine or if you want to take it to another level, I would highly recommend this book. Pavel is the Russian genius who introduced kettle bells to the Western world. His routine is far more comprehensive than mine and will loosen and strengthen your joints. A must- read if you still want to feel good in your later years.

"Super Body, Super Brain" by Michael Gonzalez-Wallace. There has been a lot of discussion over the last decade about the mind-body connection. This book will give you an additional option for mini-workouts that will not only strengthen your muscles, but will also make you more aware of how your body works and improve your balance.

"The War of Art" by Steven Pressfield. This is not a book about exercise. This is a book about getting started. For a lot of people that is the hardest part. If you feel like you can't get into shape because of whatever your reason could be, go buy this book immediately. Most people are their own worst enemy and this book will help you get past that.

"Healing Back Pain: The Mind Body Connection" by Dr. John E. Sarno. Many people won't start exercising due to chronic back pain. I have suffered with back pain myself for many years. Dr. Sarno explains how the mind can cause pain as a way to not focus on things that might be causing them mental anguish. It is one of the most influential books I have ever read. I heard about on the Howard Stern show. Howard has talked about how this book saved his life on many occasions. Please give it a read if you suffer from back pain.

"Awaken the Giant Within" by Anthony Robbins. Once again, this is not a fitness book. Many people don't try to get into shape because they have underlying issues that prevent them from trying to help themselves. If you can't picture yourself in good shape, you probably won't do the things it takes to get there. This book will help you to visualize yourself as someone who is worthy of being in shape and also to picture yourself as already accomplishing that goal.

"Can't Hurt Me" by David Goggins. There may be times in your life where you may feel sorry for yourself and that can prevent you from doing the things you know you should do. Reading this book will smack all of those thoughts right out of your head! The biggest takeaway from this book is that the extreme things this man had to overcome will keep you from feeling sorry for yourself. This man looks at doing extreme exercise as a way to toughen up your mind and help make you a better person.

Podcasts:

Below is a list of guests that have been on the Joe Rogan Experience with the episode number. Some of the people are nutrition experts, while the others ones are more motivational. Many of his guests have their own podcasts, so if Joe's not your cup of tea do some exploring on your own. To make it easier to decide which ones you might want to listen to I put an (E) for educational and an (I) for inspiration.

Ben Greenfield #1120 and #1069 (E)

Zack Bitter #1110 (E)

Peter Attia #1108 (E)

Chris and Mark Bell #1101 (E)

David Goggins #1080 and #1212 (I)

Nina Teicholz #1058 (E)

Dr. Rhonda Patrick #1054 (E)

Dr. Shawn Baker #1050 (E)

C.T. Fletcher #1044 (I)

Chris Kresser #1037 (E)

Dom D'Agostino #994 (E)

Kelly Brogan #968 (E)

Robb Wolf #935 (E)

Diamond Dallas Page #1166 (E and I)

This should be enough to get you more educated on health and fitness than 99% of your peers! Take the time to listen if you can because it will definitely help to keep you motivated. Most of these people have their own podcasts and Instagram pages you can follow for your daily motivation. As always, keep looking for new information. We live in an exciting time and there are always new things you can learn to help improve your quality of life!